SpringerBriefs in Fire

Series editor

James A. Milke, College Park, USA

More information about this series at http://www.springer.com/series/10476

Karen F. Deppa · Judith Saltzberg

Resilience Training for Firefighters

An Approach to Prevent Behavioral Health Problems

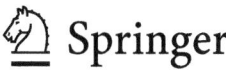 Springer

Karen F. Deppa
Brookeville, MD
USA

Judith Saltzberg
University of Pennsylvania
Wynnewood, PA
USA

ISSN 2193-6595 ISSN 2193-6609 (electronic)
SpringerBriefs in Fire
ISBN 978-3-319-38778-9 ISBN 978-3-319-38779-6 (eBook)
DOI 10.1007/978-3-319-38779-6

Library of Congress Control Number: 2016940323

© The Author(s) 2016
This work is subject to copyright. All rights are reserved by the Publisher, whether the whole or part of the material is concerned, specifically the rights of translation, reprinting, reuse of illustrations, recitation, broadcasting, reproduction on microfilms or in any other physical way, and transmission or information storage and retrieval, electronic adaptation, computer software, or by similar or dissimilar methodology now known or hereafter developed.
The use of general descriptive names, registered names, trademarks, service marks, etc. in this publication does not imply, even in the absence of a specific statement, that such names are exempt from the relevant protective laws and regulations and therefore free for general use.
The publisher, the authors and the editors are safe to assume that the advice and information in this book are believed to be true and accurate at the date of publication. Neither the publisher nor the authors or the editors give a warranty, express or implied, with respect to the material contained herein or for any errors or omissions that may have been made.

Printed on acid-free paper

This Springer imprint is published by Springer Nature
The registered company is Springer International Publishing AG Switzerland

This SpringerBrief is dedicated to fire service emergency responders everywhere—a selfless, devoted group of public servants who deserve unwavering admiration and respect for their efforts and sacrifices.

Acknowledgments

The authors acknowledge with gratitude their families, for their steady support and encouragement throughout the preparation of this brief. Karen Deppa thanks Roy, Janetta, Nate, and Garrett. Judith Saltzberg thanks Steve and Noah and also Karen Reivich, a leader in the field of resilience training and my colleague and friend for the last 25 years. Special appreciation goes to Michael A. Donahue for his reviews, suggestions, and dedication to making resilience training for firefighters a reality. Finally, a salute to the faculty and students of the University of Pennsylvania's Master of Applied Positive Psychology program for providing the resources, rigor, and perspectives that helped to lay the foundation for this report.

Contents

1	**Introduction and Statement of Goals**	1
	References	2
2	**Firefighter First Responders**	3
	2.1 The Fire Service Culture	8
	2.2 How Behavioral Health Issues in the Fire Service Have Been Approached	9
	References	13
3	**Positive Psychology: An Introduction**	17
	References	21
4	**Resilience: Dealing with Adversity and Setbacks**	23
	4.1 Optimism: A Primary Driver of Resilience	24
	4.2 Not to Be Confused with Post-traumatic Growth	25
	4.3 The Hope Circuit: Learning About Control Promotes Resilience	26
	4.4 Resilience Skills Are Teachable	27
	4.4.1 Teaching Resilience Skills to School-Age Populations	28
	4.4.2 Teaching Resilience Skills to Adult Populations	29
	References	32
5	**Major Factors that Influence Behavioral Health in the Fire Service**	35
	5.1 Thinking Patterns that Lead to Unproductive Emotions and Behaviors	35
	5.2 Relatedness, Belonging, and the Role of Social Support	38
	5.3 Perceived Coping Self-efficacy	39
	5.3.1 Stress: A Threat or a Challenge?	40
	5.3.2 Mindsets Are Malleable	41

		5.3.3	Mindsets About Stress Relate to Coping Self-efficacy	42
		5.3.4	Perceived Coping Self-efficacy in Studies Involving Emergency Responders	45
	References			48
6	**Discussion**			51
	6.1	Sample Interventions		53
		6.1.1	Interventions to Increase Realistic Optimistic Thinking	54
		6.1.2	Interventions to Increase the Quality of Social Interactions	55
		6.1.3	Interventions to Increase Coping Self-efficacy	56
		6.1.4	Measurement Tools	56
	6.2	The Case for Universal Training		58
		6.2.1	Implementation and Cultural Considerations	59
		6.2.2	Moving Toward a More Resilient Fire Service	60
	6.3	Limitations of This Review		61
	6.4	Future Directions		62
	6.5	Supplement		63
		6.5.1	Identifying ABCs—A Foundational Skill to Build Resilience	64
		6.5.2	Identifying Thinking Traps and Getting FAT Thinking	65
		6.5.3	Countering Unproductive Thoughts in Real Time	66
		6.5.4	Hunting the Good Stuff	67
		6.5.5	Active-Constructive Responding	68
		6.5.6	Building High-Quality Connections (HQCs)	69
	References			70
7	**Conclusion**			75
	Reference			76
Glossary of Terminology				77

Chapter 1
Introduction and Statement of Goals

Firefighter emergency responders routinely face work-related stresses. Violent, graphic incidents are a well-documented but unavoidable part of the job (Fisher and Etches 2003; Meyer et al. 2012). So, too, are the risks for behavioral health problems associated with those stresses (Sliter et al. 2014; Wilmoth 2014). Researchers have studied the factors associated with the development of psychological distress in this population. They have sought to find patterns and predictors pointing to when such problems are more likely to occur. Since the terrorist attacks of September 11, 2001, attention to treating psychological symptoms in emergency responders has gained greater prominence. A number of programs and guidance documents focus on addressing symptoms once they occur, or on trying to reduce the impact of events after the fact. These crucial efforts need to continue.

However, very few studies address the idea of actively trying to prevent, or at least mitigate, the negative reactions to traumatic stress *before* the exposure to events occurs. This e-book begins to fill that void by exploring the concepts and science of positive psychology. This relatively new field offers tools for learning psychological resilience, the process of adapting in a positive way to situations involving adversity or risk (Masten et al. 2009). Resilience is a default reaction for most people. But when circumstances hinder our natural ability to act in resilient ways, resilience can be fostered through a set of teachable skills. This Brief reviews factors that lead to resilience and programs that have successfully developed resilience in a variety of audiences. Based on this review, the goal of avoiding or at least reducing behavioral health problems in firefighter emergency responders seems achievable. Thus, the application of resilience training for firefighters and ultimately the development of resilient fire department environments appear to be not only feasible, but essential.

Emergency responders pledge to serve their communities in ways and to an extent that few are willing or able to do. The approach explored in this Brief capitalizes on the best aspects of the profession and culture of the fire and emergency services. In doing so, it lights a path to a more efficient and effective fire service, as well as to strengthening the coping resources of the dedicated men and women who are sworn to protecting life, property, and the environment.

References

Fisher, P., and Etches, B. (2003, October). *A comprehensive approach to workplace stress and trauma in fire-fighting: A review document prepared for the International Association of Firefighters 17th Redmond Symposium.*

Masten, A. S., Cutuli, J. J., Herbers, J. E., and Reed, M. J. (2009). Resilience in development. In S. J. Lopez and C. R. Snyder (Eds.), *Oxford handbook of positive psychology* (2nd ed., pp. 117-131). New York, NY: Oxford University Press, Inc.

Meyer, E. C., Zimering, R., Daly, E., Knight, J., Kamholz, B. W., and Gulliver, S. B. (2012). Predictors of posttraumatic stress disorder and other psychological symptoms in trauma-exposed firefighters. *Psychological Services, 9*(1), 1-15.

Sliter, M., Kale, A., and Yuan, Z. (2014). Is humor the best medicine? The buffering effect of coping humor on traumatic stressors in firefighters. *Journal of Organizational Behavior, 35*(2), 257-272.

Wilmoth, J. A. (2014, May-June). Trouble in mind. Special report: Firefighter behavioral health. *NFPA Journal.* Quincy, MA: National Fire Protection Association. Retrieved from http://www.nfpa.org/newsandpublications/nfpa-journal/2014/may-june-2014/features/special-report-firefighter-behavioral-health. Accessed 27 Feb 2016.

Chapter 2
Firefighter First Responders

As of 2013, the most recent year for which data are available, the United States was protected by approximately 30,000 fire departments. Nearly 2500 of these departments were all career, protecting primarily communities of 25,000 people or more. Almost 20,000 were all volunteer, typically protecting communities of fewer than 25,000 people. The remainder were departments that staffed a combination of career and volunteer responders, known as "combination" departments (U.S. Fire Administration 2015a). Of the estimated 1,140,750 firefighters in 2013, about 31 % were career firefighters, and 69 % were volunteers (Haynes and Stein 2014).

In addition to fighting fires and providing services related to preventing fires (such as fire investigation, fire inspection/code enforcement, fire prevention/public education), many fire departments offer specialized emergency responder services. These include vehicle extrication, wildfire/wildland urban interface protection, technical rescue, and hazardous materials response (U.S. Fire Administration 2015b). Approximately 60 % of fire departments also offer their communities some degree of emergency medical service (EMS) at a basic or advanced level (Haynes and Stein 2014). In fire departments that also provide emergency medical response, calls for medical aid constitute about 80 % of the total number of responses. Thus, in many communities, firefighters are truly our nation's first responders: first to arrive on the scene of an incident, and first to administer care to victims. A common reference to the fire department as the agency of "first and last resort" in its community highlights the all-hazard response role it plays.

This readiness comes at a cost. Firefighting was named 2015's "most stressful job in the U.S." by the career information site CareerCast, with enlisted military personnel coming in second (CareerCast 2015). This is not particularly surprising, since from the time that the first organized fire companies were established at the urging of Benjamin Franklin in Philadelphia in the 1730s, firefighters have run toward danger when most everyone else runs away from it.

Firefighters are exposed to levels of danger and both physical and psychological stress that are uncommon to most occupations (International Association of Fire

Chiefs 2015). Michael Perry, a volunteer firefighter from Wisconsin, coined an unofficial motto of the firefighter when he said, "Your worst day is our everyday" (*Into the Fire* 2006). In the course of their normal duties, they may be exposed to hazards including fire-related death and injuries, structural collapse, vehicle accidents en route to incidents, and exposures to contaminants from products of combustion, hazardous materials, and medical emergencies. Firefighters also are first on the scene in the aftermath of natural disasters, terrorist attacks, mass casualties, and environmental catastrophes. In their role as first responders, they are exposed in a very graphic way to deaths, auto accidents, child abuse, domestic violence, murders, suicides, and similar tragedies.

Workplace stresses can include overtime, the unpredictability of shift work, long hours away from home, departmental politics, interrupted sleep, the necessity of being on high alert while at work, lack of regular meals, the emotional burden of having to report tragic news, and excessive workload (Fisher and Etches 2003; Meyer et al. 2012; Milen 2009; Sivak 2016). They could be called directly from one traumatic incident to attend another one (Dowdall-Thomae et al. 2012). Volunteer firefighters serving rural areas and small communities often respond to calls involving friends and relatives, which adds a personal element to a traumatic incident (Jahnke et al. 2014). Career firefighters in one city may serve as volunteers in another city, providing an added level of exposure (Sivak 2016). The stress of the job often gets carried home and affects spouses, significant others, and other family members (Regehr 2005). Firefighters are also not immune to the everyday stressors that everyone faces, and stress at home can compound the stress experienced at work (Regehr 2005, 2009; Regehr et al. 2005). These stresses can build over time, wearing away at a firefighter's resistance, until a traumatic incident serves as a tipping point (Avsec 2016).

Firefighters are highly trained for the physical aspects of their job. This attention to training, combined with more sophisticated firefighting techniques and improved personal protective equipment, makes the job of firefighting safer than it used to be from a physical standpoint. The 10-year average of firefighter line-of-duty deaths in the United States has been steadily dropping since 2008. From 1995–2008, the yearly average of on-duty deaths was in the low 100s, and is currently at an average 83 deaths for the years 2005–2014 (Fahy et al. 2015). Still, the fact that the rate of firefighter injuries on the fireground has remained fairly steady from 1981–2014 (averaging about 25 injuries per 1000 fires) emphasizes the hazardous nature of the job (Haynes and Molis 2015).

The psychological toll of emergency response gets less attention than the physical toll, and its effects have not been as well documented. Most people are familiar with the term "mental health." However, professionals dealing with the psychological concerns affecting emergency responders refer to them as "behavioral health" issues. Behavioral health addresses the mental and emotional aspects of wellness. In addition, behavioral health addresses habits, substance use and abuse, and other physical manifestations of, and environmental contributions to, mental and emotional states.

Behavioral health problems among first responders stemming from the stresses that they face can take many forms. Some of the most common are absenteeism, burnout, depression, sleep disturbances, anxiety, alcoholism, substance abuse, and post-traumatic stress disorder (Sliter et al. 2014; Wilmoth 2014). Kaufmann et al. (2013) compared the prevalence of behavioral health problems in firefighters, police, and other protective services workers (PSWs) with workers in other occupations at baseline and over a three-year follow-up period. They found that the lifetime prevalence of mental health problems was similar between the two groups at baseline. However, during follow-up measurements, researchers found that PSWs were more likely to experience a larger variety of potentially traumatic events. Such circumstances are associated with increased risk of developing new mental and alcohol-use disorders. Because this association was particularly strong for PSWs early in their careers, researchers recommended instruction in coping skills and timely intervention for early-career PSWs to prevent future behavioral health problems (Kaufmann et al. 2013).

Posttraumatic stress disorder (PTSD) is considered a trauma- and stressor-related disorder by the 5th edition of the Diagnostic and Statistical Manual of Mental Disorders (American Psychiatric Association 2013). According to this edition, PTSD can be triggered by exposure to actual or threatened death, serious injury, or sexual violation, either by:

- Directly experiencing the traumatic event;
- Directly witnessing the traumatic event;
- Learning that the traumatic event occurred to a close family member or friend; or
- Experiencing first-hand exposure to the negative details of the event in a repeated or extreme way.

Certainly, firefighter first responders experience some or all of these exposures. Behavioral symptoms accompanying PTSD include:

- Re-experiencing the event;
- Avoidance of distressing reminders of the event;
- Having negative thoughts and mood that can comprise a range of feelings and behaviors; and
- Arousal, which includes behaviors that are destructive to self or others, sleep problems, extreme vigilance, and similar "fight or flight" responses.

Rates of current PTSD among firefighters differ according to the source of the information. Some studies (e.g., Wagner et al. 1998) report rates for a current PTSD diagnosis ranging from 18–37 %. Other studies using more rigorous diagnostic procedures report current PTSD rates from 5–13 % in the firefighting population, which is comparable to the rate of PTSD in the general population (Meyer et al. 2012).

PTSD incidence has been associated with other symptoms in German professional firefighters, including depression, social dysfunction, substance abuse, and physical complaints (Wagner et al. 1998). A study found that disaster workers exposed to a tragic airplane crash were diagnosed with higher rates of acute stress disorder, depression, and PTSD compared to a control group. These symptoms were more likely if the disaster workers were young and unmarried, had high exposure during the event, or had previous experience with disasters (Fullerton et al. 2004).

Suicide among firefighters in the United States has been a subject of attention in recent years. Suicides of high-profile members of the fire service and "clusters" of suicides among firefighters in large fire departments have caused particular alarm (Wilmoth 2014). Quantifying the prevalence of suicide in connection with firefighting compared with the general level in the population, however, has been difficult for a number of reasons. Primary among these reasons is the fact that death certificates do not always reflect that the victim was a firefighter, particularly in the case of volunteer or retired firefighters. As a result, reliable statistics on the topic historically have not been available (Gist et al. 2011). However, the Census of Fatal Occupational Injury database reveals that between 2003 and 2010, the major occupation with the highest rate of workplace suicides was Protective Service Occupations. PSWs, including firefighters, experience suicides at 5.3 suicides per 1 million, compared with the national average of 1.5 suicides per 1 million people (Tiesman et al. 2015). Thus, workers in protective service occupations are 3.5 times more likely to commit suicide on the job than the average U.S. worker.

The Firefighter Behavioral Health Alliance (FFBHA) has been collecting and validating voluntary confidential reports on firefighter suicide each year since 2012 (www.ffbha.org). The figures reported on the FFBHA site (79 in 2012; 69 in 2013; 109 in 2014; 112 in 2015) are thought to represent only about a third of the actual numbers of firefighter suicides that occur each year (Sivak 2016). If suicide in the fire service were the same as the rate in the general population, fire departments are three times more likely to experience a suicide than a line of duty death in a given year (National Fallen Firefighters Foundation 2014).

Suicidal thoughts or ideations are associated with depression, anxiety, substance abuse, PTSD, and alcohol dependence, and tend to increase the more such stressors are present (Gist et al. 2011). A study of about 1000 career, volunteer, and retired firefighters who completed a mental health survey online identified several risk factors associated with the likelihood of having experienced suicide ideation (thoughts), plans, attempts, and non-suicidal self-injury (Stanley et al. 2015). These risk factors include having a lower rank within the department and fewer years of service (generally younger firefighters), being in an all-volunteer department, being a member of a department providing EMS as well as firefighting services, being active-duty military, receiving a cancer diagnosis, and having responded to either a suicide attempt or a suicide death (Stanley et al. 2015). In this study, over 15 % of respondents reported having attempted suicide at least once while they served in the fire service. Nearly 47 % of survey respondents reported suicide ideation during their fire service career. Twenty percent reported having made a suicide plan during their career; and over 16 % reported having inflicted non-suicidal self-injury while serving as a firefighter (Stanley et al. 2015). These rates are significantly higher than the lifetime rates found among U.S. adults for the same activities. These findings prompted the researchers to call for further studies that replicate and confirm the results beyond the convenience sample used in this analysis (Stanley et al. 2015). The statistics are alarming taken in isolation, but a possible explanation of the high percentages is that respondents may have been more interested in taking the online survey because they were struggling or had struggled with mental health issues.

Retirement, particularly recent retirement, is also a risk factor in suicide among firefighters. Almost one-quarter of the 146 retiree suicides in the Firefighter Behavioral Health Alliance database occurred within the first week of retirement (Sivak 2016). Fire department membership can be all-consuming, providing an identity and a meaningful occupation or volunteer pursuit, as well as a social life. When retirement forces that activity to disappear or be drastically reduced, the psychological toll it takes on the retiree can be difficult to endure (IAFF Behavioral Wellness Manual n.d.; M. Donahue personal communication July 10, 2015).

Gist et al. (2011) suggest that the Interpersonal Theory of Suicide (Van Orden et al. 2010) is a useful way of understanding why suicides occur and in approaching interventions that have the goal of reducing suicide. The theory proposes that three

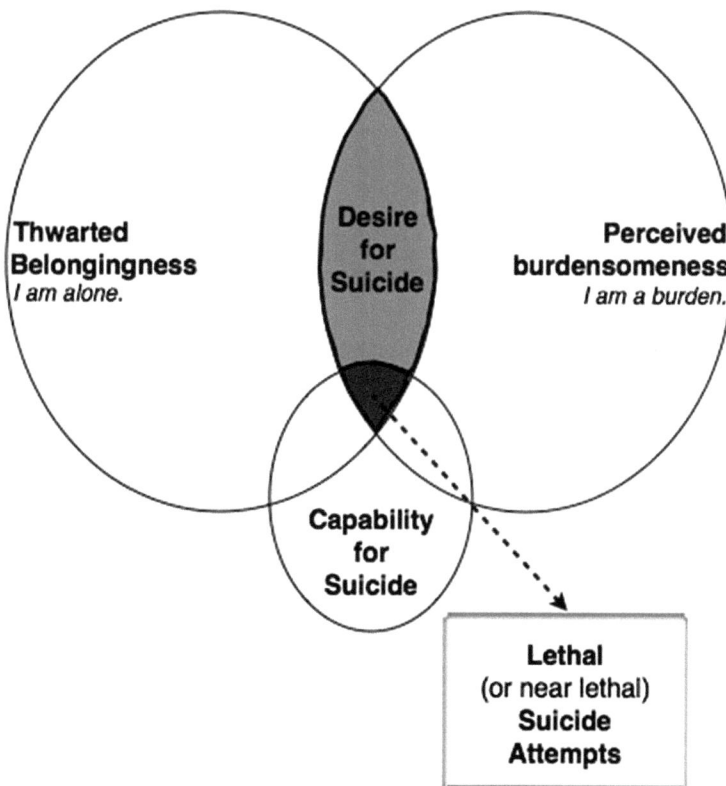

Fig. 2.1 Assumptions of the interpersonal theory of suicide (Van Orden et al. 2010). Copyright © 2010 by the American Psychological Association. Reproduced with permission

factors must be present in order for suicidal thoughts to translate into suicidal behavior. First, the individual feels social isolation from an obstructed sense of belongingness. Next, the individual perceives that he or she is a burden. Finally, the individual has the capability to engage in suicidal behavior, which is separate from the desire to do so. The dimensions of perceived burdensomeness are feeling unwanted, expendable, and an onus on others, combined with a strong sense of self-hatred. Capability comprises not only the physical means of carrying out a suicide, but a reduced fear of death and an increased tolerance for physical pain (Van Orden et al. 2010). See Fig. 2.1 for assumptions of the Interpersonal Theory of Suicide.

2.1 The Fire Service Culture

The culture of the U.S. fire service is closely linked to its history. Tradition in the fire service is a sacred concept. Tradition has its positive aspects. For example, tradition holds that firefighter emergency responders are a close-knit alliance of men and women who are service-oriented and willing to sacrifice for the greater good of their community. They share a unique camaraderie developed not only from responding to incidents together but also from drilling and training together, from sharing common experiences, both good and bad, and from living and dining together during their shifts. They look out for one another and take care of their own; they consider themselves a family. This sense of belongingness extends beyond on-duty hours. Firefighters often socialize with each other when off-duty, which serves to strengthen bonds and reinforces cultural norms (M. Donahue personal communication July 10, 2015). This cohesiveness is crucial to their ability to work together seamlessly during an incident, and creates a strong sense of belonging when not responding to emergencies as well (Marsar 2013).

But tradition also has its downsides, and the negative aspects of the firefighter culture may be contributing to an increase in preventable firefighter deaths and injuries (International Association of Fire Chiefs 2015). Though firefighter safety and health has improved over the years, many firefighters still believe that in order to be effective, they have to be fast in getting to the fire at all costs, and take personal and collective risks to get as close to the fire as possible. This "hero mentality" can perpetuate incorrect and unsafe methods of fighting fires because they are viewed as traditions (International Association of Fire Chiefs 2015). Many firefighters were indoctrinated to have an expectation that they would be injured or die while responding to incidents (M. Donahue personal communication July 10, 2015).

Dark expressions of humor about traumatic events—often referred to as "gallows humor," "black humor" or "cynical humor"—are a universal coping mechanism among emergency responders. Researchers have found that humor fulfills several functions in situations where emotions in response to adverse events might otherwise be unbearable. Expression of humor is associated with increased pain tolerance, stress relief at both the physical and emotional levels, and prevention of professional burnout (Rowe and Regehr 2010).

The use of such humor is not restricted to the helping professions. However, it is used by emergency responders within their peer interactions to reframe stressful experiences, enabling them to distance themselves from the emotions of a situation so that they can focus on managing the incident and completing necessary tasks (Rowe and Regehr 2010). Sharing this form of humor among themselves also allows firefighters to strengthen the cohesion of their group and increase social support from colleagues (Rowe and Regehr 2010). A study of career firefighters in a large Midwestern U.S. city found that a sense of humor acted as a buffer between exposure to traumatic incidents and symptoms of burnout and PTSD (Sliter et al. 2014). The researchers suggested that humor is a form of active coping—that is, coping that involves using one's own resources to deal with a problem. Humor serves to increase social bonding, promotes relaxation, and helps to reframe the adverse situation in order to make it seem less negative and stressful (Sliter et al. 2014).

On the other hand, a culture of "laughing off" traumatic incidents and other problems can be taken as discouraging someone from seeking help (M. Donahue personal communication July 10, 2015). In general, because the fire service is such a tight-knit community, outsiders and those who do not conform tend to be excluded from life in the fire station, and external influences tend to be resisted (International Association of Fire Chiefs 2015). For example, emergency responders may be reluctant to share the details of the day when they return home, in hopes of preventing distress in family members and significant others or because it is felt that they would not understand. However, this reluctance can end up distancing and isolating them from a key source of support (M. Donahue personal communication July 10, 2015).

A 2015 report on the need to create a greater safety orientation within the fire service pointed out that the features of the fire and emergency service culture that are most highly valued need not be compromised in the process of shifting the culture. Rather, changes in practice are more likely to be successful if they take the form of small adjustments rather than large, sudden transitions (International Association of Fire Chiefs 2015).

2.2 How Behavioral Health Issues in the Fire Service Have Been Approached

The traditional image of the firefighter as the strong, silent hero has fostered resistance to acknowledging and seeking out treatment for behavioral health problems. This has contributed to a lack of focus in many fire departments on mental health issues (Jahnke et al. 2014). The earliest approach to firefighter behavioral health, if it can be called an approach, involved denying that emotional and psychological problems existed at all. Firefighters were told to "suck it up," and not admit or discuss their difficulties. If they acknowledged that they were troubled, they were subject to social sanctions, such as being avoided, ignored, or ridiculed for being weak or unfit for the job (Sweeney 2014).

The stigma attached to admitting emotional and psychological vulnerability remains a problem in the fire service, and is one of the negative cultural legacies of the past. Admitting to being affected by an event directly flies in the face of the cultural image of toughness. A core belief prevails: *We are problem solvers. We don't need help; we're the ones who provide help* (M. Donahue personal communication July 10, 2015).

From the 1980s until the past decade, the most popular method for addressing responses to traumatic incidents in fire departments was the Critical Incident Stress Management (CISM) model, which featured the Critical Incident Stress Debriefing, or CISD (Regehr 2001). CISD, one element of a comprehensive crisis response program, is a structured small-group storytelling setting. CISD includes a required single-session group meeting in which participants describe the traumatic event and their reactions to it in graphic detail in an attempt to process what happened (Mitchell n.d.). The popularity of CISD has waned over the past decade in light of empirical research that questioned its effectiveness. Anecdotal reviews of CISD were reported to be positive. However, controlled studies have shown either no effect on reducing the incidence of post traumatic stress disorder or in some cases found the process to have a negative effect on some participants. This could be as a result of exposure to the traumatic reactions of others in the group (Regehr 2001). Because post-incident interactions among peers often serve as natural debriefings of traumatic events, Jahnke et al. (2014) have speculated that the mandatory group debriefing prescribed by CISD interrupts that natural process.

The developer of the CISM model has argued that the studies that are critical of CISD were poorly done. He points out that the effectiveness of the CISM program depends on properly following CISM standards and using well trained providers (Mitchell 2004). Despite the doubts that have been raised about its effectiveness, many fire departments still support the CISM model, and either manage their own team or have access to a regional CISM team (for example, Massachusetts offers access to 16 teams statewide through the Massachusetts Peer Support Network).

In the past decade, the fire service has placed more emphasis on the need for solid empirical findings of benefit to justify the resources devoted to their deployment. An action item in the 2nd National Fire Service Research Agenda, spearheaded by the National Fallen Firefighters Foundation and involving representatives from more than 50 fire service and affiliated organizations, called for additional research to identify, develop, deliver, and evaluate evidence-based tools and approaches to address firefighter behavioral health. The report cited concern that "practices lacking empirical support or even contraindicated by solid empirical evidence have been found in common usage while evidence-supported practices and techniques are not always recognized or employed" (National Fallen Firefighters Foundation 2011, p. 34).

2.2 How Behavioral Health Issues in the Fire Service Have Been Approached

Since September 11, 2001, and particularly in recent years, fire service leaders and public health professionals have teamed up to develop programs to address firefighter behavioral health issues. Many of these programs are sponsored by the major national fire service organizations. In addition, organizations have been formed specifically to raise awareness or treat behavioral health problems in fire and rescue personnel. For example:

- The National Fallen Firefighters Foundation (NFFF) has been a leader in developing its Everyone Goes Home® initiative to prevent firefighter line-of-duty deaths and injuries. Of the program's 16 Firefighter Life Safety Initiatives, number 13 is "Firefighters and their families must have access to counseling and psychological support." Among other activities to promote this initiative, the Foundation has developed an Occupational Stress Exposure Recommended Protocol for dealing with potentially traumatic events (National Fallen Firefighters Foundation n.d.). NFFF also provides training in Stress First Aid (SFA), to return fire and rescue personnel to health and readiness following a negative stress reaction. SFA leverages collaborative peer support within a department to help firefighters and providers of emergency medical services to assist each other when stress-related reactions occur, prevent the stress reactions from progressing, and connect those who need more formal treatment with appropriate care (Watson et al. 2015).
- The International Association of Fire Fighters and the International Association of Fire Chiefs are preparing updated, broader recommendations on firefighter behavioral health, including suicide prevention and awareness, as part of their Fire Service Joint Labor Management Wellness-Fitness Initiative (International Association of Fire Fighters n.d.).
- The National Fire Protection Association's NFPA® 1500 Standard on Fire Department Occupational Safety and Health Program is in the process of being updated and includes chapters on "Behavioral Health and Wellness Programs" and "Occupational Exposure to Atypically Stressful Events" (National Fire Protection Association 2015).
- The National Volunteer Fire Council, through its Share the Load™ support program, provides firefighters and emergency medical service providers with access to resources and information to assist first responders and their families in managing and overcoming problems at work and at home (National Volunteer Fire Council n.d.). The Council also offers a Fire/EMS Helpline for first responders and their families to seek help on behavioral health issues (http://www.nvfc.org/hot-topics/fire/ems-helpline).
- The Code Green Campaign (http://codegreencampaign.org/) aims to increase awareness of, and to reduce, behavioral health issues in first responders. The website publishes anonymous stories of first responders' behavioral health struggles in an effort to reduce the stigma associated with mental health issues and enable others facing similar challenges to see that they are not alone. The campaign also educates first responders on how to get help if they need it, and how to identify problems in their peers.

- The Firefighter Behavioral Health Alliance (http://www.ffbha.org/FBHA_Page.php) raises awareness about behavioral health issues in the fire service by maintaining a database for documenting firefighter suicides. The Alliance also provides behavioral health workshops to emergency responders and their families, and offers support to surviving family members of firefighter and EMS suicide victims.

In addition, many fire departments have their own peer support programs or have access to peer support networks that take advantage of help from those who share similar backgrounds and experiences, to provide an outlet for behavioral health concerns and to provide a liaison to licensed care providers if needed. Firefighters can also seek behavioral health assistance from Employee Assistance Programs (also known as Behavioral Health Assistance Programs) offered through their employers or unions, and from fire department chaplains (Fig. 2.2).

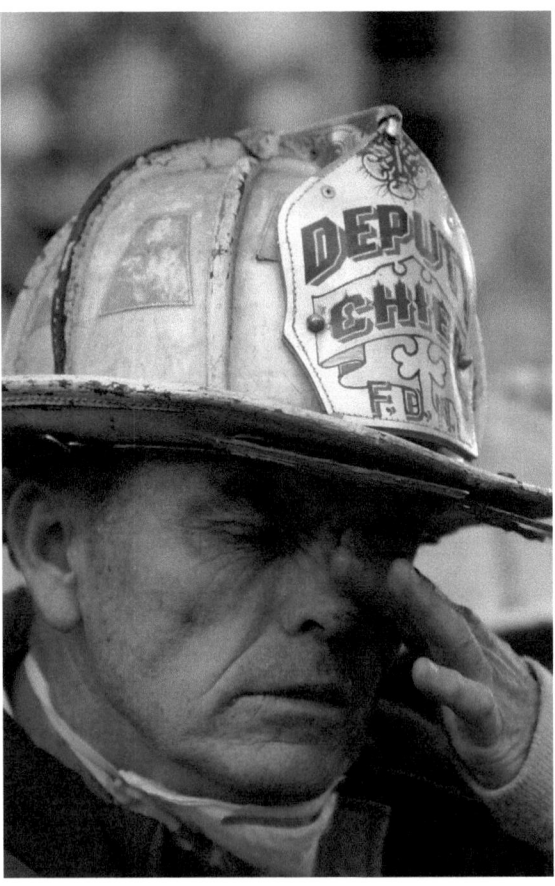

Fig. 2.2 Creative Commons Fireman-81876 by tpsdave, https://pixabay.com, licensed under CC0, public domain

These programs, and others like them, are important resources. They should continue and their results should be documented, because they address a need that has too long gone unrecognized. These programs generally take a secondary or tertiary prevention approach—that is, they address the problems *after* the critical event has taken place or the adverse reaction has occurred, and attempt to reduce their impact.

Research with fire service populations and others, which will be reviewed in this Brief, suggests that a primary prevention approach could supplement the good and important work that is already being conducted to address fire service behavioral health issues. The purpose of this approach is to strengthen the psychological resources and mental toughness of firefighters to prevent behavioral health problems *before* they occur. This is where the relatively new field of positive psychology can make an important contribution.

References

American Psychiatric Association (2013). *PTSD Fact Sheet*. Arlington, VA: American Psychiatric Publishing, Inc.

Avsec, R. (2016). Roundtable: How to fix firefighter PTSD. *Fire Chief Digital 2*(1), 7-11.

CareerCast (2015). *The most stressful jobs of 2015*. http://www.careercast.com/jobs-rated/most-stressful-jobs-2015. Accessed 27 Feb 2016.

Dowdall-Thomae, C., Gilkey, J., Larson, W., and Arend-Hicks, R. (2012). Elite firefighter/first responder mindsets and outcome coping efficacy. *International Journal of Emergency Mental Health, 14*(4), 269-281.

Fahy, R. F., LeBlanc, P. R., and Molis, J. L. (2015). *Firefighter fatalities in the United States - 2014*. Quincy, MA: National Fire Protection Association.

Fisher, P., and Etches, B. (2003, October). *A comprehensive approach to workplace stress and trauma in fire-fighting: A review document prepared for the International Association of Firefighters 17th Redmond Symposium*.

Fullerton, C. S., Ursano, R. J., and Wang, L. (2004). Acute stress disorder, posttraumatic stress disorder, and depression in disaster or rescue workers. *American Journal of Psychiatry, 161*(8), 1370-1376.

Gist, R., Taylor, V. H., and Raak, S. (2011). *White paper: Suicide surveillance, prevention, and intervention measures for the U.S. fire service*. Baltimore, MD: National Fallen Firefighters Foundation.

Haynes, H. J. G., and Molis, J. L. (2015). *U.S. firefighter injuries - 2014*. Quincy, MA: National Fire Protection Association.

Haynes, H. J. G., and Stein, G. P. (2014). *U.S. fire department profile*. Quincy, MA: National Fire Protection Association.

International Association of Fire Chiefs (2015). *National safety culture change initiative: Study of behavioral motivation on reduction of risk-taking behaviors in the fire and emergency service*. Retrieved from www.ffsafetyculture.org

International Association of Fire Fighters, AFL-CIO-CLC (n.d.). *Behavioral health*. https://www.iaff.org/HS/wfiresource/BehavioralHealth/behavioralhealth.html. Accessed on 27 Feb 2016.

Into the Fire [Motion picture on DVD]. (2006). Novato, CA: Fireman's Fund Insurance Company.

Jahnke, S. A., Gist, R., Poston, W. S. C., and Haddock, C. K. (2014). Behavioral health interventions in the fire service: Stories from the firehouse. *Journal of Workplace Behavioral Health, 29*(2), 113-126.

Kaufmann, C. N., Rutkow, L., Spira, A. P., and Mojtabai, R. (2013). Mental health of protective services workers: Results from the National Epidemiologic Survey on Alcohol and Related Conditions. *Disaster Medicine and Public Health Preparedness, 7*(01), 36-45.

Marsar, S. (2013). Camaraderie in the firehouse. http://www.firefighternation.com/article/professional-development/camaraderie-firehouse. Accessed 27 Feb 2016.

Meyer, E. C., Zimering, R., Daly, E., Knight, J., Kamholz, B. W., and Gulliver, S. B. (2012). Predictors of posttraumatic stress disorder and other psychological symptoms in trauma-exposed firefighters. *Psychological Services, 9*(1), 1-15.

Milen, D. (2009). The ability of firefighting personnel to cope with stress. *Journal of Social Change, 3*(1), 38-56.

Mitchell, J. T. (n.d.). Critical incident stress debriefing (CISD). North American Fire Fighter Veteran Network, http://www.firefighterveteran.com/images/stories/power_point/mitchell CriticalIncidentStressDebriefing.pdf. Accessed 27 Feb 2016.

Mitchell, J. T. (2004). *Crisis intervention and critical incident stress management: A defense of the field.* International Critical Incident Stress Foundation.

National Fallen Firefighters Foundation (n.d.). Psychological support. *Everyone Goes Home® 16 Firefighter Life Safety Initiatives.* http://www.everyonegoeshome.com/16-initiatives/13-psychological-support/. Accessed 27 Feb 2016.

National Fallen Firefighters Foundation (2011). *Report of the 2nd National Fire Service Research Agenda Symposium, May 20-22, 2011, National Fire Academy.*

National Fallen Firefighters Foundation (2014). Confronting suicide in the fire service: Strategies for intervention and prevention. http://www.everyonegoeshome.com/wp-content/uploads/sites/2/2015/02/Confronting_Suicide_FINAL.pdf. Accessed 27 Feb 2016.

National Fire Protection Association (2015). *NFPA 1500: Standard on Fire Department Occupational Safety and Health Program.* http://www.nfpa.org/codes-and-standards/document-information-pages?mode=codeandcode=1500andtab=about. Accessed 27 Feb 2016.

National Volunteer Fire Council (n.d.). Share the Load™ support program for fire and EMS. http://www.nvfc.org/hot-topics/share-the-load-support-program-for-fire-and-ems. Accessed 27 Feb 2016.

Regehr, C. (2001). Crisis debriefing groups for emergency responders: Reviewing the evidence. *Brief Treatment and Crisis Intervention, 1*(2), 87-100.

Regehr, C. (2005). Bringing the trauma home: Spouses of paramedics. *Journal of Loss and Trauma, 10*(2), 97-114.

Regehr, C. (2009). Social support as a mediator of psychological distress in firefighters. *The Irish Journal of Psychology, 30*(1-2), 87-98. doi:10.1080/03033910.2009.10446300

Regehr, C., Dimitropoulos, G., Bright, E., George, S., and Henderson, J. (2005). Behind the brotherhood: Rewards and challenges for wives of firefighters. *Family Relations, 54*(3), 423-435.

Rowe, A., and Regehr, C. (2010). Whatever gets you through today: An examination of cynical humor among emergency service professionals. *Journal of Loss and Trauma, 15*(5), 448-464.

Sivak, C. (2016). Why firefighters take their own lives. *Fire Chief Digital 2*(1), 4-6. http://online.fliphtml5.com/jncs/vsfx/#p=1. Accessed 27 Feb 2016.

Sliter, M., Kale, A., and Yuan, Z. (2014). Is humor the best medicine? The buffering effect of coping humor on traumatic stressors in firefighters. *Journal of Organizational Behavior, 35*(2), 257-272.

Stanley, I. H., Hom, M. A., Hagan, C. R., and Joiner, T. E. (2015). Career prevalence and correlates of suicidal thoughts and behaviors among firefighters. *Journal of Affective Disorders,* 187, 163-171.

Sweeney, P. (2014). *When serving becomes surviving: PTSD and suicide in the fire service.* http://www.crisisresponse.org/When-Serving-Becomes-Surviving-3A-PTSD-and-Suicide-in-the-Fire-Service/. Accessed 27 Feb 2016.

Tiesman, H. M., Konda, S., Hartley, D., Menéndez, C. C., Ridenour, M., and Hendricks, S. (2015). Suicide in US workplaces, 2003–2010: A comparison with non-workplace suicides. *American Journal of Preventive Medicine, 48*(6), 674-682.

References

U.S. Fire Administration (2015a). *Firefighters and fire departments.* http://www.usfa.fema.gov/data/statistics/. Accessed 27 Feb 2016.

U.S. Fire Administration (2015b). *National Fire Department Census quick facts.* https://apps.usfa.fema.gov/census/summary. Accessed 27 Feb 2016.

Van Orden, K. A., Witte, T. K., Cukrowicz, K. C., Braithwaite, S. R., Selby, E. A., and Joiner Jr, T. E. (2010). The interpersonal theory of suicide. *Psychological Review, 117*(2), 575-600.

Wagner, D., Heinrichs, M., and Ehlert, U. (1998). Prevalence of symptoms of posttraumatic stress disorder in German professional firefighters. *American Journal of Psychiatry, 155*(12), 1727-1732.

Watson, P. J., Taylor, V., Gist, R., Elvander, E., Leto, F., Martin, B., ... Litz, B. (2015). *Stress first aid for firefighters and emergency medical services personnel.* National Fallen Firefighters Foundation, Emmitsburg, MD.

Wilmoth, J. A. (2014, May-June). Trouble in mind. Special report: Firefighter behavioral health. *NFPA Journal.* Quincy, MA: National Fire Protection Association. http://www.nfpa.org/newsandpublications/nfpa-journal/2014/may-june-2014/features/special-report-firefighter-behavioral-health.

Chapter 3
Positive Psychology: An Introduction

The events of September 11, 2001, marked the beginning of a shift in how firefighter behavioral health issues are recognized and addressed. Just three years prior, in 1998, another revolution was initiated: that of a new branch of psychology known as *positive psychology*. In his inaugural address as newly elected president of the American Psychological Association, Seligman (1999) called for "a new science of human strengths" focusing on "what makes life most worth living."

The new direction toward living the best life possible was intended to supplement, not replace, the focus on repairing mental illness and suffering under the traditional disease model that characterized so-called mainstream psychology research and practice to that point (Seligman and Csikszentmihalyi 2000). A commitment to the scientific method puts positive psychology on a par scientifically with clinical psychology. This commitment also differentiates positive psychology from self-help approaches and certain branches of psychology (such as humanistic psychology) that cover similar topics but do not share an insistence on demonstrating an empirical basis for their findings and interventions (Peterson 2006).

Three main topics characterize the study of positive psychology. Positive subjective experience deals with positive emotions such as happiness and pleasure. Positive personality comprises subjects such as character strengths, virtues, and interests. Positive institutions address groups of people as they connect in communities, families, congregations, businesses, and other formal and informal organizations (Peterson 2006; Seligman and Csikszentmihalyi 2000).

As a field of study, positive psychology focuses on scientific research into the mechanisms of positive human emotions and strengths, such as joy, optimism, and courage, as well as measuring and documenting the benefits of these emotions and strengths. As a field of practice, it focuses on the application and measurement of *interventions* (that is, actions performed with the intention of bringing about change) to increase well-being, life satisfaction, physical health, and other conditions that lead to human thriving at the individual or group levels. Psychologist Christopher Peterson, one of the founders of the field, summarized the essence of positive psychology and the quest for a fulfilling life in the oft-quoted phrase, "Other people matter" (Peterson 2006, p. 249).

The theories, themes, and concepts referenced in the study of positive psychology go back to ancient times and have roots in philosophy as well as psychology. For example, Aristotle wrote that people should seek true virtue and fulfillment of human potential and excellence (which he called *eudaimonia*) above all else. For Aristotle, living eudaimonically entailed the control of self (Melchert 2002), as well as voluntarily living a reflective life guided by reason (Ryan et al. 2008). Some theorists and researchers make a distinction, as did Aristotle, between *hedonic* and *eudaimonic* well-being. Hedonic well-being refers to positive emotions, pleasure, self-gratification, and the absence of pain and distress, while eudaimonic well-being refers to the satisfaction coming from cultivating the best in oneself and realizing a deeper purpose and meaning in life (Baumeister et al. 2013; Huta 2014; Ryan et al. 2008).

Philosopher and psychologist William James wrote about "healthy-mindedness" as a tendency to regard all things as good, and noted that this tendency could be either an involuntary proclivity or it could be cultivated deliberately and systematically through habit (James 1902). Viktor Frankl (1985), writing about his experiences as a prisoner during the Holocaust, observed that his fellow prisoners who survived the concentration camps tended to be the ones who retained their optimism, hope, meaning, and the courage to carry on despite the hardships they endured. This is similar to many prisoner-of-war stories, in which the prisoners not only survive, but maintain morale and sanity in horrific situations. Faith, sense of humor, love for family, courage, integrity, honor, hope, and imagination are among the strengths POWs have called on to enable them to endure (Wong n.d.).

While positive psychology grew from a separate tradition than humanistic psychology, the celebrated psychologist Abraham Maslow and his fellow humanists in the mid-20th century promoted motivation, creativity, peak experiences and other concepts related to optimal human functioning. Maslow called this *self-actualization* (Gleitman et al. 2011).

The topics of scientific study covered under the umbrella of positive psychology include many that were conceived subsequent to the founding of the field in 1998. The creation of a space called "positive psychology" also established a unifying home for topics that had been studied earlier and that fit well into an overall science of human flourishing. For example, it was in the 1960s that Csikszentmihalyi (1990) first observed and began to study *flow* as a pathway to fulfillment in life. Flow is a state of optimal engagement and immersion in which a person controls and directs attention toward an activity, matching skills with the challenges undertaken, so that the self grows more complex. Flow states have been correlated with peak athletic performance (Jackson et al. 2001). Flow states are also associated with enhanced performance at work. Organizational resources such as social support and personal resources such as self-efficacy both facilitate and are enhanced by work-related flow (Salanova et al. 2006).

An example of a more recent topic under the positive psychology umbrella is the trait of *grit*, defined as passion for a long-term goal and perseverance toward achieving that goal despite setbacks (Duckworth et al. 2007). High grit scores are associated with greater academic achievement, and predicted higher performance in the National Spelling Bee as well as completion of a rigorous training program at West Point (Duckworth et al. 2007).

Seligman's own emphasis on the positive side of psychology grew from his development of a theory of *learned helplessness*, which he studied early in his career as a psychology researcher in the 1960s along with colleague Steven Maier. Learned helplessness was a phenomenon first observed in dogs that did not try to get away from escapable shock after experiencing inescapable shock. Seligman theorized that the dogs learned that their efforts to escape were ineffective. He later reformulated the theory to apply to humans. In humans, learned helplessness manifests as depression based on a belief that one's actions do not make a difference (Seligman 2006).

In seeking to prevent or reverse the condition of learned helplessness, Seligman pursued research on the phenomenon that he called *learned optimism*. This concept holds that one can learn and master the ability to look at situations positively, and choose to use that technique and dispute pessimistic thoughts when appropriate (Seligman 2006). For example, an optimistic explanatory style would describe misfortune as temporary, specific to that event, and caused by external events or situations. Good fortune tends to be explained by optimistic thinkers as permanent, applicable to all situations, and a result of one's own influence (Seligman 2006).

Seligman's theory of well-being evolved from the concept of learned optimism. According to Seligman's theory, well-being results from a combination of contributing factors commonly known as the PERMA model: Positive emotion, Engagement, positive Relationships, Meaning, and Accomplishment (Seligman 2011). Each of these elements is fundamental to Seligman's model. In addition to contributing to well-being, each is pursued for its own sake, rather than as a means to achieve any of the other elements in the model. Further, each can be defined and measured independently of the other elements (Seligman 2011). More recently, Seligman has agreed that vitality, or some form of physical health and fitness, is an appropriate addition to the PERMA model (M. Seligman private communication October 16, 2015).

One of the foundational concepts of positive psychology is the identification and use of character strengths. This concept studies and emphasizes the aspects of our personality that are our aptitudes for thinking, feeling, and behaving to the benefit of ourselves and others (VIA Institute on Character 2015). Character strengths are considered universal qualities that manifest themselves through thoughts, emotions, choices, and behaviors (Niemiec 2013). An early project in the history of positive psychology was the identification and classification of 24 character strengths that are thought to be substantially stable, universal qualities and that provide a common language for describing what is best in people (Peterson and Seligman 2004). All 24 character strengths are considered present in everyone to a greater or lesser degree. Those strengths that come most naturally are considered "signature strengths."

However, any of the strengths can be developed and applied individually or in combination as a pathway to greater levels of well-being (Peterson and Seligman 2004).

To name just a few of the many benefits associated with some of the well-known theories promoted under the heading of positive psychology:

- Ryff's eudaimonic model of psychological well-being includes six key elements of self acceptance, positive interpersonal relationships, autonomy, environmental mastery, purpose in life, and a mindset of personal growth (Ryff and Singer 2002). Research on women above age 60 found that those with higher scores on measures of eudaimonic well-being showed lower levels of stress, lower levels of inflammation response, more favorable cardiovascular indicators, and better quality of sleep than those with lower eudaimonic well-being. Most of these benefits were found not to correlate with high levels of hedonic well-being in the same population (Ryff et al. 2004).
- Self-determination Theory (Ryan and Deci 2000) holds that well-being results from satisfaction of the basic psychological needs of competence, autonomy, and relatedness. Competence relates to the sense of efficacy one feels in relation to his or her environment. Autonomy concerns a feeling that one's behavior is regulated by choice. Relatedness refers to feelings of connection to others. For example, feelings of competence lead to greater positive emotions or feelings. The strong sense of security in interpersonal relationships that characterizes relatedness bears heavily on a person's motivation to explore, assimilate new experiences, and develop mastery of his or her environment (Ryan and Deci 2000). Ryan et al. (2008) point out that Aristotle's concept of eudaimonia, or virtuous living, can be explained through Self-determination Theory. They assert that people who live eudaimonically tend to behave in more prosocial ways. Further, four motivational concepts drive eudaimonic living. First is the pursuit of intrinsic (internally motivated) goals and values such as relationships, health, and personal improvement for their own sake, as opposed to extrinsic (externally motivated) goals like money, power, and fame. Second comes behaving autonomously rather than in controlled, involuntary ways. Third, we find being mindful and acting mindfully. Fourth is satisfying the basic, universal psychological needs for competence, autonomy, and relatedness. Living the first three concepts helps to achieve the fourth (Ryan et al. 2008).
- The Broaden and Build Theory of Positive Emotions states that experiencing certain positive emotions (such as joy, love, and contentment) serves to broaden one's attention, thought processes, and actions, aid in problem solving, and build one's physical, social, and intellectual resources (Fredrickson 2001). For example, positive emotions have been correlated with greater psychological resilience as measured by a faster return to baseline levels of cardiovascular activity following a stressful task (Tugade and Fredrickson 2004). Through this mechanism, positive emotions are thought to have an "undoing effect" on the lingering physiology of negative emotions and on the physiology of resultant anxiety, fear, and distress (Fredrickson et al. 2000).

Positive in the context of positive psychology does not simply mean the absence of the negative. Seligman (2011) observed that in his career as a therapist treating depressed patients, he would sometimes succeed in ridding patients of the sadness, anxiety, and anger that fueled their depression. However, in the end, he did not succeed in creating happy individuals. Rather, he created "empty" patients (Seligman 2011, p. 54). Individuals who were successfully treated for depression were brought to a neutral point, but were not aware of how to create a fulfilling life or a life of optimal functioning, which required a different set of skills.

Positive psychology practitioners are often quick to point out that positive psychology is not to be dismissed as "happyology." Putting a "smiley face" on every situation is not what positive psychology is about. Beliefs that are excessively optimistic (rather than rooted in reality) can impede the ability to cope effectively and falsely convince people that they do not have to take action to avoid negative consequences (Gillham et al. 2008). Nor is positive psychology about denying things that should justifiably make us sad, anxious or angry. Indeed, seeking a balance may be the best path. Research shows (Baumeister et al. 2013) that while happiness and meaningfulness in life are positively correlated, it is possible to be high in meaning but unhappy, in part because meaningful pursuits tend to increase stress and anxiety, even when they are contributing to society and helping others. Likewise, shallowness and selfishness tend to characterize a happy life that is low in meaning (Baumeister et al. 2013).

Pawelski (2014) points out the need to consider that positive and negative states coexist in life. Negative emotions can lead to positive outcomes, and vice versa. Emotions, whether positive or negative, can have both benefits and costs. A good life takes place in a context that includes negative aspects, and dealing effectively with those negative aspects may help to define a good life. Thus, how one attends to and deals with the negative experiences that occur in a full life is, Pawelski (2014) suggests, arguably a necessary topic of study in positive psychology.

References

Baumeister, R. F., Vohs, K. D., Aaker, J. L., and Garbinsky, E. N. (2013). Some key differences between a happy life and a meaningful life. *The Journal of Positive Psychology*, *8*(6), 505-516.

Csikszentmihalyi, M. (1990). *Flow: The psychology of optimal experience*. New York, NY: Harper Perennial.

Duckworth, A. L., Peterson, C., Matthews, M. D., and Kelly, D. R. (2007). Grit: Perseverance and passion for long-term goals. *Journal of Personality and Social Psychology 92*(6), 1087-1101.

Frankl, V. E. (1985). *Man's search for meaning* (revised and updated). New York, NY: Washington Square Press.

Fredrickson, B. L. (2001). The role of positive emotions in positive psychology: The Broaden-and-Build Theory of positive emotions. *American Psychologist, 56*(3), 218-226. doi:10.1037//0003-066X.56.3.218.

Fredrickson, B. L., Mancuso, R. A., Branigan, C., and Tugade, M. M. (2000). The undoing effect of positive emotions. *Motivation and Emotion, 24*(4), 237-258.

Gillham, J. E., Brunwasser, S. M. and Freres, D.R. (2008). Preventing depression in early adolescence: The Penn Resiliency Program. In J. R. Z. Abela and B. L. Hankin (Eds.), *Handbook of depression in children and adolescents* (pp. 309–332). New York, NY: Guilford Press.

Gleitman, H., Gross, J., and Reisberg, D. (2011). *Psychology* (8th ed.). New York, NY: W. W. Norton and Company.

Huta, V. (2014). Eudaimonia. In S. A. David, I. Boniwell, and A. Conley Ayers (Eds.), *The Oxford handbook of happiness* (pp. 201-213). Oxford, UK: Oxford University Press.

Jackson, S. A., Thomas, P. R., Marsh, H. W., and Smethurst, C. J. (2001). Relationships between flow, self-concept, psychological skills, and performance. *Journal of Applied Sport Psychology, 13*(2), 129-153. doi:10.1080/104132001753149865.

James, W. (1902). *The varieties of religious experience.* Project Gutenberg Ebook. http://www.gutenberg.org/files/621/621-pdf.pdf?session_id=3282da0a9eb7d3d24a34c9772ab172ff553e66c1. Accessed 27 Feb 2016.

Melchert, N. (2002). *The great conversation: A historical introduction to philosophy* (4th ed.). Boston, MA: McGraw-Hill.

Niemiec, R. M. (2013). VIA character strengths: Research and practice (The first 10 years). In H. H. Knoop and A. Delle Fave (Eds.), *Well-being and cultures: Perspectives on positive psychology* (pp. 11-30). New York, NY: Springer.

Pawelski, J. O. (2014). *Defining the "positive" in positive psychology.* Unpublished manuscript. Philadelphia, PA: University of Pennsylvania.

Peterson, C. (2006). *A primer in positive psychology.* New York, NY: Oxford University Press.

Peterson, C., and Seligman, M. E. P. (2004). *Character strengths and virtues: A handbook and classification.* New York: Oxford American Press and Washington DC: American Psychological Association.

Ryan, R. M. and Deci, E. L. (2000). Self-determination theory and the facilitation of intrinsic motivation, social development, and well-being. *American Psychologist, 55*(1), 68-78.

Ryan, R. M., Huta, V., and Deci, E. L. (2008). Living well: A self-determination theory perspective on eudaimonia. *Journal of Happiness Studies, 9*(1), 139-170.

Ryff, C. D., and Singer, B. (2002). From social structure to biology: Integrative science in pursuit of human health and well-being. In C. R. Snyder and S. J. Lopez (Eds.), *Oxford handbook of positive psychology* (pp. 541-555). New York, NY: Oxford University Press.

Ryff, C. D., Singer, B. H., and Love, G. D. (2004). Positive health: Connecting well-being with biology. *Philosophical Transactions of the Royal Society B, 359*, 1383-1394. doi:10.1098/rtsb.2004.1521.

Salanova, M., Bakker, A. B., and Llorens, S. (2006). Flow at work: Evidence for an upward spiral of personal and organizational resources. *Journal of Happiness Studies, 7*(1), 1-22.

Seligman, M. E. P. (1999). The president's address. In *APA 1998 Annual Report, American Psychologist,* August, 1999. https://ppc.sas.upenn.edu/sites/ppc.sas.upenn.edu/files/APA%20President%20Address%201998.docx. Accessed 27 Feb 2016.

Seligman, M. E. P. (2006). *Learned optimism: How to change your mind and your life.* New York, NY: First Vintage Books.

Seligman, M. E. P. (2011). *Flourish.* New York, NY: Atria Paperback.

Seligman, M. E. P., and Csikszentmihalyi, M. (2000). Positive psychology: An introduction. *American Psychologist, 55*(1), 5-14. doi:10.1037//0003-066X.55.1.5.

Tugade, M. M., and Fredrickson, B. L. (2004). Resilient individuals use positive emotions to bounce back from negative emotional experiences. *Journal of Personality and Social Psychology, 86*(2), 320-333.

VIA Institute on Character (2015). *VIA offers personality assessment focusing on character strengths.* http://www.viacharacter.org/www/Character-Strengths/Personality-Assessment#nav. Accessed 27 Feb 2016.

Wong, P. T. P. (n.d.) Positive psychology of POW survival. International Network on Personal Meaning. http://www.meaning.ca/archives/archive/art_pos-psychology-POW_P_Wong.htm. Accessed 27 Feb 2016.

Chapter 4
Resilience: Dealing with Adversity and Setbacks

Positive psychology has identified resilience as key to the way healthy individuals handle adversity and setbacks. Resilience is about the way people deal with negative experiences that occur as part of a full life. The fire service is familiar with the term *resilience* in the context of communities and the nation's infrastructure, referring to their ability to adapt to changing conditions as well as to withstand and recover promptly from emergencies arising from manmade or natural causes (Presidential Policy Directive PPD-8 2011). In the context of positive psychology, resilience refers to the process by which individuals adapt in a positive way during or after stressful situations that involve adversity or risk (Masten et al. 2009).

Research in resilience began by studying children in the 1960s and 1970s, when it was observed that some children not only did well, but also flourished despite situations or risks in their environments or within themselves. Such situations and risks caused other children to perform poorly, lose hope, and give up. Until the term "resilient" was adopted, children in these circumstances were referred to as "stress-resistant" and even "invulnerable" by some researchers (Masten et al. 2009).

Positive adaptation (also referred to as competence) in the resilience research has proceeded on two generally accepted assumptions (Masten et al. 2009). One, that the individual is doing well in regard to behavioral expectations for their age and situation (not necessarily excelling in comparison to others). Two, the individual has been exposed in a significant way to adverse situations (which might occur in combination and accumulate over time) such that the prospect of doing well comes under serious threat. Both the positive adaptation and the exposure to risk are considered crucial to the definition of resilience (Luthar and Cicchetti 2000). Adversities can acutely or chronically disrupt normal adaptive functioning. Adversities can also hinder the development of systems that allow for adaptive functioning (Yates and Masten 2004).

Resilience can be defined by the lack of negative outcomes as well as by the presence of positive outcomes (Peterson and Seligman 2004). Factors that *moderate* (influence the strength of the relationship between) adversities and outcome in order to produce positive outcomes are known as promotive and protective factors.

These are assets, resources, and other factors, both internal and external, that work in favor of the individual to predict good adaptation and more favorable outcomes (Masten et al. 2009). Factors that moderate the adversities and the outcome such that negative outcomes are more possible are referred to as risk factors and vulnerabilities (Masten et al. 2009; Yates and Masten 2004). Promotive and protective factors, as well as risk factors and vulnerabilities, have been found to be additive, and to interact with one another (Peterson and Seligman 2004). Rutter (1987) emphasizes the importance of not just identifying vulnerabilities and protective factors, but also of understanding the mechanisms and processes behind them—that is, why they have the effects that they have in given situations.

A crucial point to keep in mind is that resilience is not a single, fixed personality trait, strength, attribute, or characteristic. Rather, resilience is a comprehensive term that refers to a series of mechanisms and processes of adapting and coping that are influenced, for better or for worse, by the interaction between assets and risks at the individual, relationship, and environmental/community levels (Garmezy 1991; Luthar and Cicchetti 2000; Yates and Masten 2004). Resilience depends on one's response to risk or adversity at a given time, in a given circumstance. An individual's ability to be resilient can change if the circumstances change (Rutter 1987). Resilience is not, therefore, a "suck it up" and "pull yourself up by your bootstraps" quality that you would have if you only tried hard enough. People demonstrate resilience to given circumstances, as opposed to being resilient as a static characteristic. Scientists and practitioners are cautioned to talk about resilient trajectories or outcomes, as opposed to resilient individuals (Luthar and Cicchetti 2000). Moreover, resilience is teachable, as will be discussed later in this chapter.

A related, essential point about resilience is that it is not a magical, heroic status that is enjoyed by a select, lucky few. Rather, resilience has been found to be a set of common, ordinary skills and adaptive processes that constitute our dominant response to dealing with hardship (Masten 2001). It is the most typical result after exposure to a potentially traumatic event (Bonanno 2005). Resilience is the result of basic human adaptive systems operating as they should. Those adaptive systems include, among other things, the ability to problem-solve, the motivation to learn and master new skills, the development of strong and secure relationships, and cultural traditions that foster opportunities for learning, mentoring, social rituals, and other adaptive activities (Masten et al. 2009). Research has found that the ability to cope is compromised more because of adaptive systems becoming overwhelmed, damaged, or undermined than because of the number or combination of risk factors (Yates and Masten 2004).

4.1 Optimism: A Primary Driver of Resilience

While several factors contribute to resilience, including ability to problem-solve, self-regulation, self-efficacy, and a sense of humor (Masten et al. 2009), researchers agree that optimism is the primary driver of resilient behavior (Reivich and

Shatté 2002). Compared with their more pessimistic counterparts, optimistic thinkers tend to persevere when faced with great challenges. They try to solve problems rather than avoiding or denying them. They find positive meaning in situations. They accept situations they cannot change but frame them in a positive perspective. They relieve distressing situations with humor. Finally, they take better care of their health and have better immune response (Carver et al. 2009).

Optimism has been defined in terms of being hopeful about future events and believing that things can change for the better. This orientation is known as dispositional optimism (Carver et al. 2009). Another definition looks at optimism in terms of explanatory style and the ability to influence events, in which optimistic thinkers are more likely to explain adverse events as external (not caused by me), temporary (this too shall pass), and specific (affecting just this situation). Optimistic thinkers tend to explain positive events as internal (I had something to do with it), permanent (this is always how it is), and pervasive (affecting everything rather than just that one situation) (Peterson and Steen 2009; Seligman 2006).

Positive psychology does not advocate blind, unquestioning optimism that is habitually and universally applied in all circumstances and at all costs. Seligman (2006) advocates a state of realistic optimism. Also known as flexible optimism, it is optimism that one can choose to apply, depending on the requirements of, and one's goals for, a given situation. Techniques that teach optimistic thinking through the use of cognitive-behavioral therapies focus on addressing negative, distorted interpretations of events and reframing them to more positive interpretations without ignoring the reality of the situation (Carver et al. 2009). To this point, researchers on resilience often refer to an adverse event as a *potentially* traumatic event (e.g., Bonanno 2005). This term recognizes that there is nothing necessarily inherent in an event itself that makes it traumatic. Rather, those who experience and interpret the event determine whether it will result in psychological distress.

4.2 Not to Be Confused with Post-traumatic Growth

Resilience is not to be confused with post-traumatic growth. Post-traumatic growth is the experience of positive psychological change and transformation as the result of struggling with traumatic life situations (Tedeschi and Calhoun 2004). Post-traumatic growth is characterized by a heightened appreciation for life, a change in priorities, greater spirituality, increased compassion, and a sense of finding meaning in suffering. Post-traumatic growth is considered an outcome of the process of coping with adversity and a desirable outcome that can help one deal with future trauma. For example, a study following new police recruits in Australia for 12 months after beginning service found that experiencing a trauma prior to joining the police force was associated with a tendency to adapt in a positive way to potentially traumatic events experienced on the job, based on their self-reported experience of post-traumatic growth (Burke and Shakespeare-Finch 2011).

A key difference between resilience and post-traumatic growth is that post-traumatic growth is not consciously pursued, and often occurs simultaneously with the distress from the adverse event. Thus, it is possible to experience both PTSD and post-traumatic growth (Tedeschi and Calhoun 2004). Studies of Israeli adolescents who experienced terrorist events and of members of the Israeli army who had participated in the second Lebanon War found that those who did not suffer from PTSD (and thus were considered resilient according to the researchers) had the lowest scores for post-traumatic growth, suggesting that resilience and post-traumatic growth are inversely related (Levine et al. 2009). It should be noted, however, that failure to develop PTSD by itself should not be considered evidence of resilience in an individual, especially when determining policy and interventions (Almedom and Glandon 2007).

4.3 The Hope Circuit: Learning About Control Promotes Resilience

Intriguing new research suggests that, contrary to Seligman's learned helplessness theory (referred to in the Chap. 3), helplessness might not be "learned" after all. Rather, it might be our default position that can only be unlearned. This research comes nearly 50 years after Seligman and Maier formulated the learned helplessness theory (Seligman 2006). This emerging understanding of helplessness and how it is prevented may have significant implications for resilience theory.

Learned helplessness theory assumed that learning that an event was uncontrollable led to negative psychological consequences and passive behaviors, which then had to be unlearned (Seligman 2006). However, research by Maier and colleagues on brain chemistry and neurochemical mechanisms in rats suggests the opposite is true. Passivity appears to be the *dominant,* default response to a stressor. But the passive response can be reversed in laboratory rats. When they learn that they have control and mastery over a situation, the rats do not become helpless. Researchers concluded that when rats learn that they have control, this knowledge suppresses the activity in the portion of the brain that would otherwise produce a passive/helpless response (Maier 2015).

A nagging unanswered question associated with learned helplessness theory was why some people exposed to a traumatic, uncontrollable stressor develop clinical problems, while others seem resistant to or recover quickly from the same stressor. In pursuing a biological explanation to this question, Maier focused on an area of the brain called the dorsal raphe nucleus (DRN). The DRN, when manipulated experimentally in the laboratory, can be activated to produce helpless behaviors in laboratory rats or inactivated to prevent helpless behaviors in rats (Maier et al. 2006). Out of the laboratory, in real-life conditions, the DRN activates by default, unless it gets a signal not to activate. An area of the brain called the ventral medial prefrontal cortex (vmPFC) inhibits the neural response of the DRN to stressors when the rat experiences control over a situation, such as an escapable shock.

The experience of control prevents the helpless behavior. Inactivating the vmPFC experimentally leads to passive behavior in rats, even in situations that allow the rats to learn escape behaviors (Maier et al. 2006).

Based on this research, Maier et al. (2006) concluded that experiences with behavioral control over situations promote resilience in rats via activation of the vmPFC. Further, this suggests that prior experiences of control and other coping activities are protective because they activate the vmPFC, which inhibits the DRN and other stress-responsive parts of the brain. This suppression effect lasts over time (Maier 2015). These findings help to explain Seligman's learned optimism theory, in which having had control over a past adverse situation makes it more likely that one will feel control over an unrelated future adverse situation (Seligman 2006).

If the mechanism can be shown to work in humans as it does for lab rats, Seligman sees tremendous implications for the future of positive psychology and the study of resilience (Seligman 2015). Seligman refers to the brain's vmPFC-DRN connection as the "Hope Circuit." The latest research suggests that developing self-efficacy, in the form of expectations of control and mastery, builds and strengthens the Hope Circuit. The Hope Circuit then activates to inhibit and overcome a default response of helplessness and passivity. The Hope Circuit, Seligman points out, is where positive psychology and resilience training have their greatest effect (Seligman 2015).

The importance of feelings of self-efficacy, including mastery and the ability to cope with adversity, to resilience in general and to firefighter emergency responder resilience in particular, will be revisited later in this Brief.

4.4 Resilience Skills Are Teachable

Prevention activities (known as *interventions*, or activities designed to bring about change and reduce risks and threats) can be divided into primary, secondary, and tertiary prevention. *Primary prevention* has the goal of preventing a negative event or reaction before it occurs. This can be done by preventing exposure to hazards, by changing behaviors that can lead to negative events (or to adverse reactions to those events), and by increasing one's resistance to negative outcomes if exposure were to take place. The aim of *secondary prevention* is to reduce the impact of a negative event that has already occurred. This is done in order to stop or slow the progression of an adverse reaction, prevent long-term problems, and return individuals to their status before the event. *Tertiary prevention* takes place after the negative event has already occurred and has produced a lasting adverse reaction. This level of prevention attempts to alleviate the long-term negative impacts of the reaction.

Researchers have studied resilience for the past five decades. However, the relatively recent development of positive psychology has encouraged a shift in emphasis in resilience research. Whereas earlier resilience research focused largely on addressing negative responses to stressful events after they occurred, more recent research concentrates on preventing the negative response in the first place. In other words, emphasis has moved from a secondary or tertiary preventive approach toward a primary preventive approach. Primary prevention is achieved through the development of defenses and the boosting of assets and resources to enable a healthy, adaptive response (Yates and Masten 2004).

Research on resilience tends to follow one or a combination of three strategies (Masten et al. 2009). Risk-focused strategies aim to reduce risks and vulnerabilities, i.e., exposure to hazardous experiences and situations. Asset-focused strategies strive to increase the number of, quality of, or access to assets and resources required for positive adaptation. Process-focused strategies center on marshaling and strengthening the basic, fundamental protective systems required for normal human development. Masten et al. (2009) note that resilience is most threatened when adversity undermines these basic protective systems.

Interventions in the realm of resilience research address three levels of functioning (Masten et al. 2009). At the level of the individual, the focus is on such skills as effective problem solving, stress response, and self-regulation. At the level of relationships, the focus includes supportive attachments to friends, family, and partners. At the level of the environment, the focus is on the surroundings in which the individuals and relationships operate. Significantly, the research literature strongly cautions against attempts to work on individual skills in isolation. The relationships and the environment in which the individual operates must also be taken into account. The most effective interventions are those that are multi-faceted, and take into account the functioning of the individual in the context of various levels of influence (Luthar and Cicchetti 2000).

The two basic takeaways from this research are that individuals are capable of learning skills that facilitate resilience, and that environments can be organized in ways that foster resilience (Gillham et al. 2014). Teaching aspects of resilient thinking and behaviors can improve coping levels and prevent depression. This is particularly true when the adversities one encounters are especially traumatic or frequent, and overwhelm the levels of resilience we normally depend on from day to day (Reivich and Shatté 2002).

Bonanno (2004) expresses concern that attempts to teach resilient responses could interrupt the natural processes that lead to improved resilience. He proposes that such interruption could end up making an individual less resilient. While this is an interesting position to consider, studies that have been done on the effects of resilience training programs for school-age and adult populations, such as those described next, do not support this conclusion. These studies appear to indicate that they have achieved many of the sought-after benefits, and have not done harm to those receiving the training.

4.4.1 Teaching Resilience Skills to School-Age Populations

Much of the research on resilience interventions has focused on school children. For example, the University of Pennsylvania designed the Penn Resiliency Program (PRP) as a group depression-prevention intervention for late-elementary and middle school students ages 10–14. Curriculum developers chose this age group for particular focus because, in most cases, first episodes of depression occur in adolescence (Gillham et al. 2008). The curriculum uses age-appropriate cognitive-behavioral interventions delivered over twelve group sessions lasting 90–120 min. The curriculum, divided into a cognitive component and a social-problem-solving component, teaches skills and techniques designed to reinforce and facilitate each other. These skills include the detection and evaluation of thinking styles, identifying inaccurate thoughts, how to dispute negative beliefs in the moment, and techniques for problem solving, negotiating, decision-making, assertiveness, and relaxation (Gillham et al. 2008).

A meta-analysis of both targeted and universal studies evaluating the PRP (Brunwasser et al. 2009) found greater levels of optimism and modest but reliably lower levels of depressive symptoms in participants through 12 months of follow up compared to controls. The reduction and prevention of depressive symptoms appeared to be more meaningful in participants with elevated baseline symptoms. Notably, the average effect size across studies showed a larger effect (in the form of fewer symptoms of depression) at a 6-month follow up than immediately after the intervention (Brunwasser et al. 2009). This delayed effect is likely due to the fact that symptoms take time to develop in those who become depressed. Further, the skills learned during the intervention improve and thus have more impact as they are practiced over time (Cutuli et al. 2013).

A high school positive psychology program developed by the same team that created the Penn Resiliency Program built on the skills taught in the PRP (Gillham et al. 2014). The high school curriculum is based on the three pathways to happiness presented by Seligman (2002): the Pleasant Life, the Engaged Life, and the Meaningful Life. The Pleasant Life module teaches ways to facilitate positive emotions with a focus on gratitude, savoring, and optimism. The Engaged Life module assists students in identifying and developing their character strengths (those that are most natural as well as those that are important to them) and using them in their everyday activities. The unit on the Meaningful Life encourages students to reflect on what makes life meaningful for them and for others. All of the modules encourage the students to apply these lessons on a daily basis and use them in fostering strong social connections with others and pursuing goals that serve a larger purpose. Preliminary results of a 4-year scientific evaluation indicate that the program did not affect students' reports of depression or anxiety. However, teachers and parents reported improvements in the students' social skills and engagement in school. Students with lower grades prior to the implementation of the program also did better academically as a result of the program (Gillham et al. 2014).

4.4.2 Teaching Resilience Skills to Adult Populations

Resilience training has also been applied to adult populations, and the U.S. military has taken two noteworthy approaches. A program called the Boot Camp Survival

Training for Navy Recruits—A Prescription (BOOT STRAP) sought to address stress, depression, situational events, interpersonal considerations, and performance among Navy recruits (Williams et al. 2004). Recruits who were determined to be "at risk" for depression (based on higher scores on the Beck Depression Inventory 2nd Edition and the Perceived Stress Scale) were placed in two groups, one receiving the intervention and one not receiving it. A control group of recruits not "at risk" was used as a comparison. Because of limited time available for training, the intervention was delivered in 45 min group sessions once weekly over the course of the 9-week recruit training. All recruits participated in weekly group sessions. However, only the intervention group received training on cognitive behavioral techniques for coping, increasing one's sense of belonging, decreasing thought distortions, and managing stress. The at-risk recruits who received the intervention reported significant increases in their sense of belonging and camaraderie with their peers by the end of the training. They also demonstrated problem-solving coping more frequently. Finally, they reported less loneliness, decreased their insecure attachments, and increased their secure attachments compared to the non-intervention group (Williams et al. 2004).

A follow up to the BOOT STRAP study, called STARS, or Strategies to Assist Navy Recruits' Success (Williams et al. 2007), applied the BOOT STRAP intervention to entire divisions of Navy recruits, not just those deemed "at risk." Eight divisions were randomly selected to receive training, which took place during basic training, and eight divisions served as control groups. During the training, recruits were encouraged to apply the skills in their own lives as well as to coach each other in using the skills. At the end of the training, the intervention divisions reported significantly higher scores on group cohesion and perceived social support measures compared to the control groups. The intervention divisions also reported lower stress levels and decreased emotional reactivity to stressors. In addition, they experienced higher problem-solving coping skills, higher perceived social support, and less conflict in relationships. Finally, their anger expression scores were lower than the control groups.

Notably, both Navy programs also had effects on retention rates. Fewer at-risk recruits who received the BOOT STRAP intervention were sent home during recruit training. Recruit training retention rates for the intervention group (84 %) were higher than for the nonintervention group (74 %) and comparable to the comparison (i.e., not at-risk) group (86 %; Williams et al. 2004). This difference was statistically significant. During a two-year period of data collection in the STARS study, the intervention divisions had a statistically significant 3.4 % lower separation from the Navy during basic training than the control group, which researchers attributed to the training. This represented 1,120 more recruits who stayed in the Navy after basic training as a result of the intervention. The cost of replacing each separated recruit, considering costs associated with recruitment and 9 weeks of basic training, was estimated to be just shy of $19,000, with the cost of the resilience training to prevent separation estimated at about $1600. The researchers calculated that the intervention could save the Navy millions of dollars by retaining more recruits and decreasing separation costs, even taking the cost of the intervention into consideration (Williams et al. 2007).

The challenges facing the volunteer fire service regarding recruitment and retention are well known even though reliable national statistics are not available regarding the extent of the problem. A volunteer who works full-time can take four months or longer to complete the 100 h Firefighter I certification, devoting several nights a week and weekends to the training, before that volunteer can respond to an incident (U.S. Fire Administration 2007). This is a substantial time period in which a department must keep a volunteer engaged and motivated to reach the most basic goal of service. Similarly, no national studies indicate the dropout rate for career recruit schools, but conservative estimates place it at about 10 percent (M. Donahue personal communication February 24, 2016). In addition, the cost of firefighter training school is substantial. For example, the 12-week Fire Recruit Academy at Texas A&M can cost upwards of $7,000 per student, taking into account tuition, personal protective equipment, uniforms, and class supplies (http://www.careerigniter.com/questions/how-much-does-firefighting-school-cost/). Thus, the potential for a resilience training program to improve fire department retention rates is an additional benefit that could save money and strengthen both career and volunteer departments' resources.

The U.S. Army is carrying out another large-scale deployment of adult resilience training based on the PRP (Reivich et al. 2011). The Master Resilience Trainer (MRT) course is a 10-day program based on a train-the-trainer model, in which resilience fundamentals are taught to noncommissioned officers, who then teach the skills to their soldiers. The four components of the MRT comprise definitions and competencies of resilience, building mental toughness, identifying and using character strengths, and strengthening relationships.

The first independent review of the effectiveness of the MRT found that soldier-reported levels of resilience and psychological health (R/PH) were significantly higher in units exposed to MRT than in control units (Lester et al. 2011). Certain dimensions of R/PH improved significantly (for example, higher emotional fitness, good coping and friendship skills, and less catastrophizing). Further, while the training appeared to be more effective for younger soldiers, there was no evidence that soldiers reported lower R/PH as a result of exposure to MRT or that they were harmed by MRT (Lester et al. 2011). A subsequent study evaluating the effectiveness of MRT in view of mental and behavioral health outcomes indicated that soldiers who had an MRT-trained sergeant in their unit were less likely to receive diagnoses for mental health problems such as anxiety, depression, or PTSD (Harms et al. 2013). This was an indirect effect that was mediated by changes in optimism and adaptability. In addition, soldiers in units exposed to MRT experienced significantly lower rates of diagnosed substance abuse than those in control units. The researchers surmise that the MRT's beneficial effects may reach beyond individual soldiers to improving the effectiveness and efficiency of the Army as an organization (Harms et al. 2013).

References

Almedom, A. M, and Glandon, D. (2007). Resilience is not the absence of PTSD any more than health is the absence of disease. *Journal of Loss and Trauma, 12*(2), 127-143.

Bonanno, G. A. (2004). Loss, trauma, and human resilience: Have we underestimated the human capacity to thrive after extremely aversive events? *American Psychologist, 59*(1), 20-28.

Bonanno, G. A. (2005). Resilience in the face of potential trauma. *Current Directions in Psychological Science, 14*(3), 135-138.

Brunwasser, S. M., Gillham, J. E., and Kim, E. S. (2009). A meta-analytic review of the Penn Resiliency Program's effect on depressive symptoms. *Journal of Consulting and Clinical Psychology, 77*(6), 1042-1054.

Burke, K. J., and Shakespeare-Finch, J. (2011). Markers of resilience in new police officers: Appraisal of potentially traumatizing events. *Traumatology, 17*(4), 52-60.

Carver, C. S., Scheier, M. F., Miller, C. J., and Fulford, D. (2009). Optimism. In C. R. Snyder and S. J. Lopez (Eds.), *Oxford Handbook of Positive Psychology* (2nd ed., pp. 303-311). New York, NY: Oxford University Press.

Cutuli, J. J., Gillham, J. E., Chaplin, T. M., Reivich, K. J., Seligman, M. E. P., Gallop, R. J., et al. (2013). Preventing adolescents' externalizing and internalizing symptoms: Effects of the Penn Resiliency Program. *The International Journal of Emotional Education, 5*(2), 67-79.

Garmezy, N. (1991). Resilience and vulnerability to adverse developmental outcomes associated with poverty. *American Behavioral Scientist, 34*(4), 416-430.

Gillham, J. E., Brunwasser, S. M. and Freres, D.R. (2008). Preventing depression in early adolescence: The Penn Resiliency Program. In J. R. Z. Abela and B. L. Hankin (Eds.), *Handbook of depression in children and adolescents* (pp. 309–332). New York, NY: Guilford Press.

Gillham, J. E., Abenavoli, R. M., Brunwasser, S. M., Linkins, M., Reivich, K. J., and Seligman, M. E. P. (2014). Resilience education. In S. A. David, I. Boniwell, and A. Conley Ayers (Eds.), *The Oxford handbook of happiness* (pp. 609-630). Oxford, UK: Oxford University Press.

Harms, P. D., Herian, M. N., Krasikova, D. V., Vanhove, A., and Lester, P. B. (2013). *The comprehensive soldier and family fitness program evaluation report #4: Evaluation of resilience training and mental and behavioral health outcomes.* Monterey, CA: Office of the Deputy Under Secretary of the Army.

Lester, P. B., Harms, P. D., Herian, M. N., Krasikova, D. V., and Beal, S. J. (2011). *The comprehensive soldier and family fitness program evaluation report #3: Longitudinal analysis of the impact of Master Resilience Training on self-reported resilience and psychological health data.* Washington, DC: Office of the Vice Chief of Staff, Department of the Army.

Levine, S. Z., Laufer, A., Stein, E., Hamama-Raz, Y., and Solomon, Z. (2009). Examining the relationship between resilience and posttraumatic growth. *Journal of Traumatic Stress, 22*(4), 282-286.

Luthar, S. S., and Cicchetti, D. (2000). The construct of resilience: Implications for interventions and social policies. *Development and Psychopathology, 12*, 857-885.

Maier, S. F. (2015). Behavioral control blunts reactions to contemporaneous and future adverse events: medial prefrontal cortex plasticity and a corticostriatal network. *Neurobiology of Stress, 1*, 12-22.

Maier, S. F., Amat, J., Baratta, M. V., Paul, E., and Watkins, L. R. (2006). Behavioral control, the medial prefrontal cortex, and resilience. *Dialogues in Clinical Neuroscience, 8*(4), 397-406.

Masten, A. S. (2001). Ordinary magic: Resilience processes in development. *American Psychologist, 56*, 227-238.

Masten, A. S., Cutuli, J. J., Herbers, J. E., and Reed, M. J. (2009). Resilience in development. In S. J. Lopez and C. R. Snyder (Eds.), *Oxford handbook of positive psychology* (2nd ed., pp. 117-131). New York, NY: Oxford University Press, Inc.

References

Peterson, C., and Seligman, M. E. P. (2004). *Character strengths and virtues: A handbook and classification.* New York: Oxford American Press and Washington DC: American Psychological Association.

Peterson, C., and Steen, T. A. (2009). Optimistic explanatory style. In C. R. Snyder and S. J. Lopez (Eds.), *Oxford Handbook of Positive Psychology* (2nd ed., pp. 313-321). New York, NY: Oxford University Press.

Presidential Policy Directive PPD-8 (2011). *National preparedness.* Washington, DC: The White House.

Reivich, K. and Shatté, A. (2002). *The resilience factor: 7 Essential skills for overcoming life's inevitable obstacles.* New York, NY: Broadway Books.

Reivich, K. J., Seligman, M. E. P., and McBride, S. (2011). Master resilience training in the U.S. Army. *American Psychologist, 66*(1), 25-34. doi:10.1037/a0021897.

Rutter, M. (1987). Psychosocial resilience and protective mechanisms. *American Journal of Orthopsychiatry, 57*(3), 316-331.

Seligman, M. E. P. (2002). *Authentic happiness: Using the new positive psychology to realize your potential for lasting fulfillment.* New York, NY: Free Press.

Seligman, M. E. P. (2006). *Learned optimism: How to change your mind and your life.* New York, NY: First Vintage Books.

Seligman, M. E. P. (2015). Positive psychology: The cutting edge in research and teaching. Keynote address, Fourth World Congress on Positive Psychology, International Positive Psychology Association, Orlando, FL, June 26, 2015.

Tedeschi, R. G. and Calhoun, L. G. (2004). Posttraumatic growth: Conceptual foundations and empirical evidence. *Psychological Inquiry, 15*(1), 1-18. doi:10.1207/s15327965pli1501_01.

U.S. Fire Administration (2007). *Retention and recruitment for the volunteer emergency services: Challenges and solutions.* Report FA-310. Washington, DC: Federal Emergency Management Association.

Williams, A., Hagerty, B. M., Yousha, S. M., Horrocks, J., Hoyle, K. S., and Liu, D. (2004). Psychosocial effects of the Boot Strap intervention in Navy recruits. *Military Medicine, 169*(10), 814-820.

Williams, A., Hagerty, B. M., Andrei, A. C., Yousha, S. M., Hirth, R. A., and Hoyle, K. S. (2007). STARS: Strategies to assist Navy recruits' success. *Military Medicine, 172*(9), 942-949.

Yates, T. M. and Masten, A. S. (2004). Fostering the future: Resilience theory and the practice of positive psychology. In P. A. Linley and S. Joseph (Eds.), *Positive psychology in practice* (pp. 521-539). Hoboken, NJ: John Wiley and Sons.

Chapter 5
Major Factors that Influence Behavioral Health in the Fire Service

Could the firefighter emergency responder population also benefit from training on resilience skills, as school-age children and military populations have? In order to investigate this and recommend an appropriate intervention strategy, this chapter looks at what the literature says about the key factors that influence firefighter behavioral health. In a review of literature that identifies vulnerabilities and protective factors associated with behavioral health in the fire and emergency services, several factors turn up repeatedly. They provide clues to the interventions that might be most effective in a resilience training approach with this population.

5.1 Thinking Patterns that Lead to Unproductive Emotions and Behaviors

The thoughts and beliefs that we have in response to events in our lives determine how we feel and behave in relation to those events. When we can accurately, thoroughly, and flexibly interpret each event, we free ourselves to respond in the most productive way (Reivich and Shatté 2002). When we develop a tendency to interpret events habitually in the same way every time, however, we lose perspective about the realities of each situation, and our responses can fall into destructive, or maladaptive, patterns (Reivich and Shatté 2002). A form of maladaptive thinking patterns that has been found to be a risk factor for psychological distress following trauma is *negative self-appraisal*, or unfavorable evaluations about oneself. These negative self-appraisals can stem from people's perfectionist expectations of themselves that they can never meet. The negative self-appraisals lead to their developing doubts about their abilities or competence (Carver et al. 2009).

A study of career firefighters from four departments in the Midwest found that those who had difficulty coping with stress also had trouble putting their concerns into perspective. Additionally, they reported a lack of social support from family members, peers, and co-workers, and had a negative outlook on their ability to succeed professionally and at life in general (Milen 2009).

In another study, trainee firefighters were initially assessed for PTSD, a history of traumatic events, and the tendency to express negative self-appraisals, and then re-assessed after 4 years. Participants who developed PTSD over the course of the study engaged in more frequent negative appraisals about themselves than participants without PTSD (Bryant and Guthrie 2007). The researchers surmised that negative self-image was intensified by the traumatic experience and helped to predict PTSD.

A study of police, fire-rescue workers, doctors, nurses and hospital workers who responded either directly or indirectly to two emergencies involving fatalities (McCammon et al. 1988) identified several impediments to recovery from trauma. These include the tendency for emergency responders to suppress their anxiety and fear not only during the incident (which may well be necessary to function in the moment), but after the incident as well. The difficulty of letting go of the emotion-free condition called "going clinical" could be a barrier to resilience and recovery (M. Donahue personal communication July 10, 2015). This tendency is further exacerbated by disillusionment stemming from the responders' own unrealistic expectations about their ability to have a positive impact on a disastrous situation (McCammon et al. 1988).

As mentioned in Chap. 2, negative self-appraisal also looms large in people who are at risk for suicide, according to the Interpersonal Theory of Suicide (Van Orden et al. 2010). The negative self-evaluation includes the perception of being a burden to others, which contains an element of self-hatred.

Other research indicates that thinking about the good that they do in their jobs can help firefighters to counteract the negative self-appraisals and other types of maladaptive thinking associated with psychological distress. Borrowing from identity theory, Lee and Olshfski (2002) suggest that a high level of commitment to the job, whether as a career or volunteer, motivates firefighters to serve their community. They commit to an identity for which they expect themselves, and others expect them, to act heroically and altruistically. A study of 156 firefighters in upstate New York, both career and volunteer, found that the firefighters' willingness to put extra effort into their jobs was correlated with their belief that the community values and supports their work (Lee and Olshfski 2002).

Beyond the mere expectation to act altruistically, prosocial behavior (behavior intended to benefit others) in firefighters has also been found to be associated with *positive affect*—the observable expression of positive emotions or feelings. In other words, helping others can make you feel good. A study of 68 career firefighters and rescue emergency responders in Switzerland, Germany, and Austria looked into the belief and judgment that one's actions on the job are helpful to others (known as perceived prosocial impact) and how that belief relates to positive affect at home, after the work day is done (Sonnentag and Grant 2012). The researchers found that perceptions of prosocial impact predicted positive affect at the end of the workday, suggesting that good experiences at work can spill over into non-work environments. Several factors accounted for that result, including positive reflections about the workday and feelings of increased perceived competence (Sonnentag and Grant 2012).

Importantly, perceived prosocial impact can also help to counteract negative self-evaluations that put one at risk for distress following trauma. In studies of professional fundraisers and public sanitation employees, Grant and Sonnentag (2010) addressed employees' negative evaluations of themselves and their work tasks. The negative evaluations are signs of low *intrinsic motivation* (that is, little or no enjoyment of the work for its own sake) and lead to emotional exhaustion, depletion of resources, and less energy on the job. One study examined professional fundraisers who focused on how the donations they collected helped others (for example, by funding scholarships for underprivileged students). The other study featured employees of a public sanitation plant who felt pride in their efforts to serve the public by providing safe and sanitary drinking water. The results of both studies suggested that employees who self-reported low intrinsic motivation and low core self-evaluations were protected from emotional exhaustion by high levels of perceived prosocial impact. The researchers found support for their hypothesis that perceived prosocial impact helps to prevent employee burnout on the job by compensating for negative evaluations of task and self.

Thus, perceived prosocial impact safeguards against feelings of being emotionally exhausted and helps to maintain high levels of job performance (Grant and Sonnentag 2010). When the employees directed their attention outward rather than on the self, the focus on the prosocial impact of their jobs prevented them from ruminating about the unpleasant aspects of their jobs. The perceived prosocial impact also resulted in positive emotion that made the employees feel more competent and valued because they helped others. The positive emotion diverted them from negative self-appraisals, and inhibited emotional exhaustion (Grant and Sonnentag 2010).

Another study asked a nationally representative sample of adults age 18 to 89 about any charitable behaviors they engaged in and determined their genetic receptiveness to the hormone oxytocin, which helps to reduce stress responses such as anxiety. Researchers followed the participants for two years, collecting data on their stressful life events and the onset of physician-diagnosed physical illnesses (such as heart problems, cancer, diabetes, and stroke). Those who had a particular receptivity to oxytocin were less likely to suffer any new ill health effects following recent stressful events when they had reported involvement in charitable behavior. Results suggested that engaging in prosocial behavior improves physical health by activating the release of oxytocin and thus buffering the negative health effects of stress. The researchers suggest that during times of great stress, helping others might be just as beneficial to health as receiving help from others (Poulin and Holman 2013).

5.2 Relatedness, Belonging, and the Role of Social Support

As mentioned in Chap. 3, a person's sense of relatedness to others is one of the three pillars of Self Determination Theory that supplies our motivation to make our way in the world (Ryan and Deci 2000). Belonging is a fundamental human need that motivates the desire to form social and interpersonal bonds with others that are pleasant and enduring. Furthermore, high degrees of belongingness strongly correlate with improved health and well-being (Baumeister and Leary 1995).

Several studies point out the importance of a supportive social environment in reducing the stress response to trauma. A study of male firefighters in one Midwestern community (Varvel et al. 2007) reported that the firefighters experienced lower levels of stress when they felt that their supervisors provided support in the form of reliable alliance (the sense of security from knowing that help is available if needed), social integration (the feeling of being part of a larger group), and reassurance of worth (in the form of positively recognizing one's skills and abilities). In a study of social workers (Boscarino et al. 2004), both job burnout and secondary trauma—trauma resulting not from direct exposure to the trauma but from working with or otherwise encountering people who are themselves traumatized—were less likely to be associated with a supportive work environment. Regehr (2009) reported on studies of firefighters in which social support was found to be an important factor in cases of work-related psychological distress. A study of Australian career firefighters found that higher levels of perceived support from spouse, family, and friends were associated with lower levels of depression. A qualitative study of Canadian firefighters also cited support from friends and family, and particularly from the management of the fire department, as protective factors in reducing stress and trauma-related reactions (Regehr 2009).

Another study examined fire recruits in Canada during their first week of employment and following a 10-week training period, compared with a group of experienced firefighters (Regehr et al. 2003). The researchers reported that, for both groups, as levels of perceived social support decreased, levels of depression and symptoms of traumatic stress increased. However, experienced firefighters reported significantly lower perceived social support from their family and employer. They also reported lower levels of self-efficacy and higher levels of depression and trauma symptoms, indicating that firefighting takes a toll psychologically over time and may make them more vulnerable to the effects of traumatic stress (Regehr et al. 2003).

Similarly, a cross-sectional study comparing stress and coping mechanisms in three groups of Australian firefighters (recruit level, on-shift, and firefighters who had experienced a traumatic situation involving a death) explored how PTSD symptoms and coping strategies evolved over the course of a firefighter's career (Chamberlin and Green 2010). The researchers reported that older age was associated with higher levels of psychological stress, but that the coping strategy of seeking support from others predicted lower levels of post-traumatic stress in all groups (Chamberlin and Green 2010). Receiving social support was related to increases in psychological well-being and post-traumatic growth, and to lower levels of PTSD incidence, in Australian emergency medical dispatchers (Shakespeare-Finch et al. 2014). A study of Italian rescue workers found that degree of life satisfaction was associated with the workers' sense of community and collective efficacy (that is, their ability to work collaboratively and effectively) within their organization (Cicognani et al. 2009).

A meta-analysis of 37 studies by Prati and Pietrantoni (2010) looked at the role of received and perceived social support among first responders. Researchers found that social support had a significant relationship to psychological health and well-being. Moreover, *perceived* social support had a greater effect size than *received* social support. Specifically, knowing the help was available if needed produced more well-being than actually seeking and receiving that help (Prati and Pietrantoni 2010).

In their study of fire and rescue personnel from a large urban department in the southern United States, Farnsworth and Sewell (2011) found that the presence of social support predicted fewer PTSD symptoms. However, negative social interactions (involving criticism, disappointment, or other unpleasant exchanges or behaviors) and fear of emotion were associated with greater levels of PTSD symptoms. Further, fear of emotion was found to account for the relationship between PTSD symptom severity for both social support and negative social interactions. The researchers found that PTSD interventions that encourage the recalling of traumatic memories are less likely to be successful in those who fear their emotions. Researchers had three suggestions for those applying PTSD interventions to consider before they ask participants to re-experience traumatic events. First, interventions should take into account how each participant processes emotions. Second, the interventions should focus on minimizing negative social interactions in addition to increasing social support. Third, interventions should incorporate treatment approaches from successful PTSD programs that provide instruction on emotional awareness and regulation, such as the positive and negative effects of anger (Farnsworth and Sewell 2011).

As noted in Chap. 2, the Interpersonal Theory of Suicide (Van Orden et al. 2010) holds that a thwarted sense of belongingness and the ensuing social isolation are among the factors that must exist for a person to want to attempt suicide.

5.3 Perceived Coping Self-efficacy

Self-determination Theory states that well-being lies in a person's ability to master the basic psychological needs of competence, autonomy, and relatedness (Ryan and Deci 2000). Self-efficacy, a concept related to competence, derives from the theoretical framework of Social Cognitive Theory, which explains human behavior in terms of agency—the capacity to explore, manipulate, and influence one's environment (Bandura 1999). Self-efficacy is the belief and confidence in one's personal agency, or ability to act in a way that brings about a desired outcome (Maddux 2009).

Self-efficacy beliefs develop from several sources. Self-efficacy is most strongly related to our own efforts to control five variables (Bandura 1982; Maddux 2009):

- our environment (performance experiences)
- what we learn from observations of others' behaviors (vicarious experiences)
- our ability to imagine how we or others would act in hypothetical situations (imaginal experiences)
- others' beliefs about our capabilities
- our physical and emotional states.

High self-efficacy has been shown to be related to happiness and well-being, less depression and anxiety, adoption of healthy behaviors, and effective immune functioning, as well as our ability to self-regulate (Maddux 2009). Self-efficacy beliefs affect people's sense of mastery, their decisions about behaviors, and their choice of activities. Higher self-efficacy scores indicate that someone will more strongly persist in his or her efforts, especially when conditions change or become challenging. Thus, self-efficacy is more influential than innate ability or talent in determining whether a person will reach his or her goals (Maddux 2009).

Self-efficacy is not just a matter of knowing what to do in a given situation, and successful performance by itself is not enough to create beliefs of self-efficacy. Self-efficacy involves people's judgments about how well they can carry out a course of action for an anticipated situation. This construct is often referred to as *perceived* self-efficacy (Bandura 1982). Individuals who judge an activity to be beyond the capacity of their ability to cope will tend to avoid that activity, will dwell on their own shortcomings, and will inflate the difficulty of future activities. These negative thoughts and behaviors lead to stress and poor performance, even if a person knows what to do in the situation (Bandura 1982).

An event can be interpreted either as a frightening threat or a surmountable challenge, depending on how confident a person feels in his or her ability to manage the event (Benight and Bandura 2004). This confidence in the ability to manage the event is known as coping self efficacy.

5.3.1 *Stress: A Threat or a Challenge?*

Coping refers to the process of evaluating a given stressor and marshaling the personal resources to deal with the stress. According to Crum et al. (2013), traditional coping strategies assume that stress is invariably harmful, and teach people that they should manage or avoid stress. Certainly, the job of the first responder is to engage actively with highly stressful situations, not to avoid them.

In summarizing the research on stress, McGonigal (2015) cites three factors that make stress most likely to have harmful effects: (1) When the stress overwhelms your ability to cope with it; (2) when the stress isolates you from others; and (3) when the stress seems to lack meaning and feels involuntary. The negative effects of stress, particularly chronic stress, are well documented (e.g., Taylor 2010) and frequently communicated in the workplace, by doctors, and through the media.

Just the belief that stress is a killer is correlated with higher mortality in individuals who report high levels of stress. In one such study (Keller et al. 2012), participants who responded to the 1998 National Health Interview Survey conducted by the National Center for Health Statistics answered specific questions on perceived stress, perceived health impacts of stress, and stress management. Those respondents who reported experiencing a lot of stress and who also believed that stress impacted their health a lot had a 43 % increased risk of premature death over the nine-year follow-up period compared with those who did not report either the stress or the negative beliefs about stress. Researchers stopped short of declaring a causal connection between perceptions of the health impacts of stress and the experience of high stress. However, they did point out that the combination could be providing a synergistic effect on the risk of premature death (Keller et al. 2012).

Not nearly as well known or as broadly communicated are the positive effects of stress. The fact that stress can lead to both good and bad effects is known as the *stress paradox*. These positive effects can include (Crum et al. 2013):

- better mental and physical functioning to meet immediate demands;
- improved initiative, problem-solving, attention, and memory;
- enhanced immunity and physical recovery;
- mental toughness; and
- the benefits that accrue with post-traumatic growth, such as enhanced appreciation for life, heightened spirituality, and a sense of meaning.

The *challenge* state in response to stress occurs when a person perceives that his or her personal resources are sufficient to meet or exceed the stress of the situation. A person experiences the *threat* state when the perceived demands of the situation are greater than the resources he or she can call upon to meet the demands (Jamieson et al. 2013). Whether we consider stress to be a challenge or a threat—that is, what our *mindset* about stress is—appears to be in large part a matter of choice.

5.3.2 Mindsets Are Malleable

Mindset refers to how we think about things. Our mindset comprises the beliefs and expectations we have that shape our reality and through which we filter our experiences. Mindsets help to guide our judgments, actions, behaviors, and even our health (Dweck 2008; Crum et al. 2013).

Brief interventions, such as a video with factual information delivered one time, can change a person's mindset about whether personal qualities like intelligence are fixed or changeable traits (Dweck 2008) and how a person views the effects of stress on health (Crum et al. 2013). Even such brief interventions can have lasting effects on mindset (Cohen and Sherman 2014). Moreover, a change in mindset can affect not only how a person thinks about a particular topic, but also how his or her body responds to those thoughts, and how well he or she performs tasks. For example:

- A study that taught housekeepers in a hotel that cleaning hotel rooms qualified as exercise changed the housekeepers' perception of themselves from non-exercisers to exercisers. This shift in perception, or mindset, regarding their perceived level of exercise, resulted in small but significant objective physical health improvements compared to housekeepers in the control group. This was the case even though both the experimental and control groups continued to perform the same amount of work and did not report differences in other habits (Crum and Langer 2007). One alternative explanation that cannot be ruled out is that although the housekeepers performed the same number of hours of work in each of the two groups, the researchers did not measure how vigorously they performed these routine tasks. Nonetheless, researchers concluded that mindset mediates (accounts for the relationship between) exercise and health.
- Another experiment looked at how changing a person's mindset affects physiological response. Researchers asked study participants to drink a milkshake at two different times. One time they were told that they were getting a sensible low-fat diet shake, and the other time, a decadent, high-calorie, high-fat shake. In reality, participants got the same exact shake both times. But their bodies reacted differently depending on what they believed they were drinking. When they believed they were getting the decadent shake, their bodies' levels of the hunger-inducing hormone grehlin dropped and made them feel more full and satisfied, compared to when they believed they were drinking the sensible shake (Crum et al. 2011).
- A study of the effect of mindset expectations on motor performance found that boosting participants' general expectations about their ability to perform well under pressure improved their accuracy compared to a control group in a high-pressure situation involving a throwing task with which they had no prior experience (McKay et al. 2012).

5.3.3 Mindsets About Stress Relate to Coping Self-efficacy

Turning attention to the specific effects of mindsets about stress, researchers explored the extent to which the mindset that stress is bad (debilitating) or good (enhancing) correlated with health consequences deriving from the experience of stress (Crum et al. 2013). Studies in which participants have a stress-is-enhancing mindset report less depression and anxiety compared to those with a stress-is-debilitating mindset. They also report higher energy levels, workplace performance, and overall life satisfaction (Crum et al. 2013).

Those with a stress-is-enhancing mindset also are more likely to cope with stress using *approach behaviors*. Approach behaviors include seeking feedback, looking for solutions, and setting goals, in order to cope with the stressful situation. People with a stress-is-debilitating mindset tend to cope using *avoidant* strategies, such as through alcohol use, withdrawal, and rumination, in an attempt to get away from or otherwise reduce the stress (Crum et al. 2013).

A stress-is-enhancing mindset appears to be positively associated with coping self-efficacy. When people gain new skills to manage challenges, self-efficacy increases. Self-efficacy also rises when people encounter new information to discredit inaccurate beliefs about their capabilities and fears (Bandura 1982). Having had the experience of successfully coping with past adversity can be a protective factor for coping with future negative events because of the resultant increase in self-efficacy (Rutter 1987). The stronger one's feeling of self-efficacy, the more likely one will be to actively address stressful situations. Consequently, one will have greater success in shaping the outcome of the situation rather than feeling controlled by the situation (Benight and Bandura 2004).

Those with a higher sense of coping self-efficacy are more solution-focused and tend to take actions and adopt strategies that shape challenging events in ways that produce better outcomes (Benight and Bandura 2004). They are more successful in part because they put more effort into meeting the challenge and do not give up as easily (Bandura 1982). Completing tasks successfully is associated not only with greater feelings of self-efficacy, but also with greater self-esteem and more positive personal relationships (Rutter 1987).

Experiments to increase coping self efficacy through a change in the stress mindset have produced promising results. Jamieson et al. (2013) studied the effects of *stress reappraisal*—that is, reinterpreting emotions, thoughts, and physical manifestations of a stressful situation in a way that changes one's mindset about stress from negative to positive. They review several studies that support the hypothesis that exercising stress reappraisal can shift the body's response during stress from negative effects to positive effects. The threat state elicits a decrease in cardiac efficiency and inhibited blood flow throughout the vascular system. The body's response to a challenge state, however, is improved blood flow and greater cardiac efficiency (Jamieson et al. 2013). Researchers found that when they instructed subjects to interpret the arousal they felt during times of acute stress as a resource to improve performance, subjects reported better outcomes than those who interpreted their arousal as harmful (Jamieson et al. 2013).

Significantly, participants were not trying to ignore, escape from, or decrease their level of arousal, but rather to change their relationship to the stress and thus their response to it while maintaining a high level of arousal. Not only did the body respond in a more adaptive way when participants were taught to reappraise their arousal, but the body also returned to pre-stress levels more quickly after the situation was over (Jamieson et al. 2013). The ability of stress/arousal reappraisal to interrupt negative appraisals of a stressful situation, and change negative outcomes to more positive ones, is depicted in Fig. 5.1.

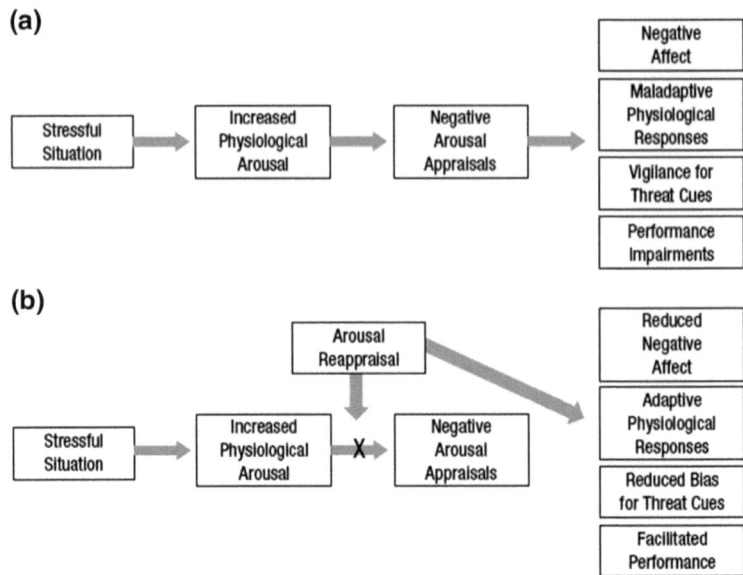

Fig. 5.1 These two panels show how stress that results in increased physiological arousal can lead to either negative appraisals and undesirable outcomes (**a**), or to more beneficial results (**b**) when the physiological arousal is reappraised to shift negative interpretations of stress to more positive ones (Jamieson et al. 2013). Copyright © 2013 by SAGE Publications. Reproduced with permission

Another cognitive behavioral technique that has been effective in increasing coping self-efficacy is the practice of writing about seeking meaning in the stressful situation. Meaningfulness tends to be associated with helping others and being oriented toward future goals, even to the point of sacrificing personal pleasures in the moment (Baumeister et al. 2013). This tie between meaning and prosocial behavior is significant to the role of firefighter emergency responders. They are not only in a unique position to help others in their darkest hours, but they have made the conscious choice to do so.

Reflecting on one's core personal values can help transform stressful experiences into meaningful experiences and improve one's ability to cope with stress (McGonigal 2015). Such reflection serves to remind people of the personal resources they can bring to the stressful situation and reduce the negative impact of the stress on well-being. Further, reflection increases the likelihood that people will deal with the stressful situation proactively and effectively, rather than through avoidance coping (Cohen and Sherman 2014). Affirming one's personal values also serves as a buffer against the negative effects of stress by encouraging reappraisal of the threatening situation, helping to keep pessimistic thoughts in check, and placing the stressful situation into a larger context of big-picture goals (Cohen and Sherman 2014).

For example, a study of women who had completed treatment for early-stage breast cancer asked the women to write about their cancer four times over a three-week period for 20 min at a time. Those who were asked to address their deepest thoughts and feelings about their cancer and those who were asked to address positive thoughts and feelings about their cancer reported less subjective distress immediately after the writing exercise. They also had fewer self-reported health problems at a 3-month follow-up compared to a control group that was asked to write about facts regarding cancer treatments (Creswell et al. 2007). Analysis of the content of the women's writings suggested that the participants who benefited the most from the intervention were those who recognized and affirmed values that were important to them, such as religion and relationships, or who wrote about personal qualities in themselves that they valued. The exercise helped them to affirm their ability to cope with adversity, to process their thoughts about their cancer in a more positive way, and to find meaning in the experience they had been through (Creswell et al. 2007).

Another study (Sherman et al. 2009) asked college students facing their most stressful college exam to complete assessments about their academic and social concerns, and to choose and rank their most important values from a list. The students in the self-affirmation portion of the experiment were asked to write for 10 min each about their top two most important values, why they were important and an important time in their life when they were able to embody the values. Compared to a control group that wrote in a general way about values that were not personally important to them, the participants who reflected on and affirmed their values in two brief writing exercises reported feeling less stress and worry during their exam period (including being less concerned about failure). In addition, the experimental group had a reduced physiological response to the stress hormone epinephrine during the exam period compared to the control group. Researchers concluded that the self-affirmation exercise served to buffer the students from the negative hormonal effects of stress on health (Sherman et al. 2009).

Choosing to see stress as a common human experience, connecting the stressful events to one's personal values, and recognizing that one's stress is connected to a larger purpose in life does not remove the stress, by any means. It does, however, make one's life more meaningful to choose to see the stress in a larger context (McGonigal 2015). This is not to say that benefits can or should be found in every stressful or traumatic event. Nor does it imply that we should force people to find the good in every horrific situation. However, the ability to see the good as well as the bad in adverse situations leads to better coping skills and a healthier response to stress in some populations. Cultivating this habit may help prevent behavioral health problems in the fire service population as well.

5.3.4 *Perceived Coping Self-efficacy in Studies Involving Emergency Responders*

Self-efficacy is often discussed in connection with specific roles, activities, or situations rather than in a global sense. Perceived coping self-efficacy has been shown to be a primary factor that accounts for recovery after a traumatic situation, as well as a protective factor against development of PTSD (Benight and Bandura 2004).

Looking specifically at studies involving emergency responders and self-efficacy, a study of Italian rescue workers (including male and female firefighters, paramedics, and medical technicians) reported that respondents high in self-efficacy tended to be less affected by conditions of high stress, compared with workers with low self-efficacy. Researchers used the Professional Quality of Life Scale, which measures levels of *compassion satisfaction*—that is, the pleasure that one gets from helping others and making a positive difference. It also measures *compassion fatigue*, also known as secondary traumatic stress, which is a lessening of compassion over time accompanied by a negative attitude and other symptoms. They found that in rescue workers with high self-efficacy scores, compassion satisfaction was not affected by stress levels. Among workers with low self-efficacy, however, compassion satisfaction was positively related to reported stress levels. These findings supported the researchers' hypothesis that self-efficacy acts as a buffer between stressful events and professional quality of life (Prati and Pietrantoni 2010).

The use of active coping strategies in a study of career and volunteer Italian firefighters and emergency medical personnel showed a positive correlation with the quality of life indicators of compassion satisfaction, sense of community, and both individual self-efficacy and collective efficacy (Cicognani et al. 2009). In the same study, avoidant coping strategies such as self-criticism and distraction were associated with higher levels of burnout and compassion fatigue. This is consistent with findings of other research that avoidance-oriented coping is related to higher levels of psychiatric and post-traumatic symptoms among first responders (Cicognani et al. 2009).

A study of Australian emergency medical dispatchers found that increases in self-efficacy were related to increases in psychological well-being. Emergency medical dispatchers can experience vicarious, or secondary, trauma from dealing with stresses such as the need to make urgent decisions about traumatic events and judge situations based on incomplete information (Shakespeare-Finch et al. 2014).

German career firefighters were tested on psychological and biological health measures immediately after basic training and periodically for two years (Heinrichs et al. 2014). Researchers reported that the number and severity of traumatic events encountered by the firefighters did not correlate with development of PTSD symptoms over the course of the 24 months. However, over the two years of the study, firefighters who exhibited high hostility levels coupled with low levels of self-efficacy at the baseline evaluation showed other signs of psychological distress. These included a significant increase in PTSD symptoms, depression, anxiety, general psychological distress, and emotional dysfunction (Heinrichs et al. 2014).

Frazier et al. (2002) conducted a literature review looking at reactions between perceived control and symptoms of post-traumatic stress. The studies they reviewed indicated that perceived control in the present (what can I do about the situation now) and in the future (can I do something to prevent this situation in the future) were associated with fewer PTSD symptoms and better overall adjustment to traumatic incidents. This is consistent with models proposing that PTSD is more likely to occur when events are perceived as uncontrollable (Frazier et al. 2002).

The Firefighter Coping Self-Efficacy Scale (FFCSE) is a 20-item self-report instrument that measures how capable the respondent feels in successfully dealing with the demands of the job. In developing the scale, Lambert et al. (2012) reported that firefighters who scored higher on perceived competence for coping with the stresses and trauma of firefighting also reported less work-related stress and fewer behavioral health problems. The researchers also found that a higher score on the FFCSE was associated with higher levels of social support and positive relationships, more self-acceptance, higher levels of perceived autonomy, a sense of mastery over one's environment, and greater purpose in life. Lower scores on the FFCSE predicted PTSD and general psychological symptoms associated with exposure to traumatic incidents (Lambert et al. 2012).

Drawing from research involving a range of subjects, Benight and Bandura (2004) propose a mechanism for the role of perceived coping self-efficacy in mitigating or preventing traumatic stress symptoms. When traumatic stress arises, it can result in a threat to and rapid depletion of one's most valued resources. These resources include tangible objects such as housing, environmental conditions such as secure work and social support, energies such as knowledge, and personal characteristics such as self-esteem and coping self-efficacy (Hobfoll 1991). This loss of resources can result in PTSD and related symptoms, but the extent to which it does (if it does at all) depends on the individual's degree of coping self-efficacy (Benight and Bandura 2004). Likewise, both social support and dispositional optimism (the belief that more good things than bad will happen in the future) are resources that have been shown to reduce the likelihood of PTSD and related symptoms. These beliefs are mediated by coping self-efficacy.

Benight and Bandura (2004) propose that degree of coping self-efficacy a person has accounts for the likelihood of resource loss to result in PTSD. In other words, the greater the coping self-efficacy, the less likely resource loss will result in PTSD and related symptoms. By the same token, the loss of resources results in PTSD symptoms to the extent that a person lacks belief that he or she is able to effectively cope with the trauma. Further, they theorize that coping-self-efficacy also accounts for the impacts of optimism and social support on their ability to alleviate PTSD and related symptoms. That is, social support and optimism reduce the likelihood and severity of PTSD symptoms because of the belief in one's capability to cope effectively. Moreover, self-efficacy not only mediates (accounts for the effect of) social support in reducing PTSD symptoms, but also is a key factor in one's ability to establish social support. Self-efficacy enables people to find, cultivate, and maintain social support (Benight and Bandura 2004). These relationships among resource loss, social support, optimism, coping self-efficacy, and PTSD symptoms are depicted in Fig. 5.2.

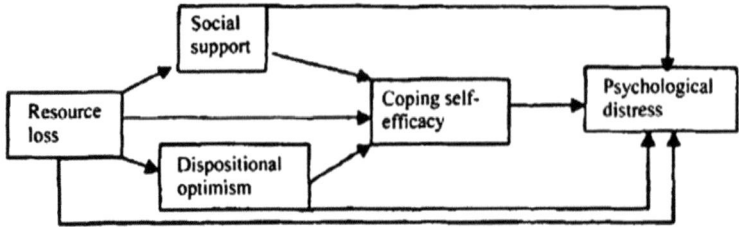

Fig. 5.2 Path analysis showing how coping self-efficacy mediates (accounts for the relationship between) resource loss and psychological stress/PTSD symptoms. Social support and optimism mediate the relationship between resource loss and coping self-efficacy (Benight et al. 1999). Copyright © 1999 by John Wiley and Sons. Reproduced with permission

Choosing to see the benefits of stress does not mean denying that stress can be harmful. However, McGonigal (2015) advocates a more balanced view of stress in which it is seen as a resource to help people engage with life and as a reaction to be trusted rather than feared.

References

Bandura, A. (1982). Self-efficacy mechanism in human agency. *American Psychologist, 37*(2), 122-147.
Bandura, A. (1999). A social cognitive theory of personality. In L. Pervin and O. John (Eds.), *Handbook of personality* (2nd ed., pp. 154-196). New York, NY: Guilford Publications. (Reprinted in D. Cervone and Y. Shoda [Eds.], *The coherence of personality*. New York, NY: Guilford Press).
Baumeister, R. F., and Leary, M. R. (1995). The need to belong: Desire for interpersonal attachments as a fundamental human motivation. *Psychological Bulletin, 117*(3), 497-529.
Baumeister, R. F., Vohs, K. D., Aaker, J. L., and Garbinsky, E. N. (2013). Some key differences between a happy life and a meaningful life. *The Journal of Positive Psychology, 8*(6), 505-516.
Benight, C. C., and Bandura, A. (2004). Social cognitive theory of posttraumatic recovery: The role of perceived self-efficacy. *Behaviour Research and Therapy, 42*(10), 1129-1148.
Benight, C. C., Swift, E., Sanger, J., Smith, A., and Zeppelin, D. (1999). Coping self-efficacy as a mediator of distress following a natural disaster. *Journal of Applied Social Psychology, 29*(12), 2443-2464.
Boscarino, J. A., Figley, C. R., and Adams, R. E. (2004). Compassion fatigue following the September 11 terrorist attacks: A study of secondary trauma among New York City social workers. *International Journal of Emergency Mental Health, 6*(2), 57-66.
Bryant, R. A., and Guthrie, R. M. (2007). Maladaptive self-appraisals before trauma exposure predict posttraumatic stress disorder. *Journal of Consulting and Clinical Psychology, 75*(5), 812-815.
Carver, C. S., Scheier, M. F., Miller, C. J., and Fulford, D. (2009). Optimism. In C. R. Snyder and S. J. Lopez (Eds.), *Oxford Handbook of Positive Psychology* (2nd ed., pp. 303-311). New York, NY: Oxford University Press.
Chamberlin, M. J. A., and Green, H. J. (2010). Stress and coping strategies among firefighters and recruits. *Journal of Loss and Trauma, 15*(6), 548-560. doi:10.1080/15325024.2010.519275.

References

Cicognani, E., Pietrantoni, L., Palestini, L., and Prati, G. (2009). Emergency workers' quality of life: The protective role of sense of community, efficacy beliefs and coping strategies. *Social Indicators Research*, *94*(3), 449-463.

Cohen, G. L., and Sherman, D. K. (2014). The psychology of change: Self-affirmation and social psychological intervention. *Annual Review of Psychology*, *65*, 333-371.

Creswell, J. D., Lam, S., Stanton, A. L., Taylor, S. E., Bower, J. E., and Sherman, D. K. (2007). Does self-affirmation, cognitive processing, or discovery of meaning explain cancer-related health benefits of expressive writing? *Personality and Social Psychology Bulletin*, *33*(2), 238-250.

Crum, A. J., and Langer, E. J. (2007). Mind-Set Matters Exercise and the Placebo Effect. *Psychological Science*, *18*(2), 165-171.

Crum, A. J., Corbin, W. R., Brownell, K. D., and Salovey, P. (2011). Mind over milkshakes: Mindsets, not just nutrients, determine ghrelin response. *Health Psychology*, *30*(4), 424-429.

Crum, A. J., Salovey, P., and Achor, S. (2013). Rethinking stress: The role of mindsets in determining the stress response. *Journal of Personality and Social Psychology*, *104*(4), 716-732.

Dweck, C. S. (2008). Can personality be changed? The role of beliefs in personality and change. *Current Directions in Psychological Science*, *17*(6), 391-394.

Farnsworth, J. K., and Sewell, K. W. (2011). Fear of emotion as a moderator between PTSD and firefighter social interactions. *Journal of Traumatic Stress*, *24*(4), 444-450.

Frazier, P., Berman, M., and Steward, J. (2002). Perceived control and posttraumatic stress: A temporal model. *Applied and Preventive Psychology*, *10*(3), 207-223.

Grant, A. M., and Sonnentag, S. (2010). Doing good buffers against feeling bad: Prosocial impact compensates for negative task and self-evaluations. *Organizational Behavior and Human Decision Processes*, *111*(1), 13-22.

Heinrichs, M., Wagner, D., Schoch, W., Soravia, L. M., Hellhammer, D. H., and Ehlert, U. (2014). Predicting posttraumatic stress symptoms from pretraumatic risk factors: A 2-year prospective follow-up study in firefighters. *American Journal of Psychiatry*, *162*(12), 2276-2286.

Hobfoll, S. E. (1991). Traumatic stress: A theory based on rapid loss of resources. *Anxiety Research*, *4*(3), 187-197.

Jamieson, J. P., Mendes, W. B., and Nock, M. K. (2013). Improving acute stress responses: The power of reappraisal. *Current Directions in Psychological Science*, *22*(1), 51-56.

Keller, A., Litzelman, K., Wisk, L. E., Maddox, T., Cheng, E. R., Creswell, P. D., and Witt, W. P. (2012). Does the perception that stress affects health matter? The association with health and mortality. *Health Psychology*, *31*(5), 677-684.

Lambert, J. E., Benight, C. C., Harrison, E., and Cieslak, R. (2012). The Firefighter Coping Self-efficacy Scale: Measure development and validation. *Anxiety, Stress and Coping*, *25*(1), 79-91.

Lee, S. H., and Olshfski, D. (2002). Employee commitment and firefighters: It's my job. *Public Administration Review*, *62*(S1), 108-114.

Maddux, J. E. (2009). Self-efficacy: The power of believing you can. In C. R. Snyder and S. J. Lopez (Eds), *Oxford handbook of positive psychology* (2nd ed., pp. 335-344). New York, NY: Oxford University Press.

McCammon, S., Durham, T. W., Allison Jr, E. J., and Williamson, J. E. (1988). Emergency workers' cognitive appraisal and coping with traumatic events. *Journal of Traumatic Stress*, *1*(3), 353-372.

McGonigal, K. (2015). *The upside of stress: Why stress is good for you, and how to get good at it*. New York, NY: Penguin Random House.

McKay, B., Lewthwaite, R., and Wulf, G. (2012). Enhanced expectancies improve performance under pressure. *Frontiers in Psychology*, *3*, 1-5.

Milen, D. (2009). The ability of firefighting personnel to cope with stress. *Journal of Social Change*, *3*(1), 38-56.

Poulin, M. J., and Holman, E. A. (2013). Helping hands, healthy body? Oxytocin receptor gene and prosocial behavior interact to buffer the association between stress and physical health. *Hormones and Behavior, 63*(3), 510-517.

Prati, G., and Pietrantoni, L. (2010). The relation of perceived and received social support to mental health among first responders: A meta-analytic review. *Journal of Community Psychology, 38*(3), 403-417.

Regehr, C. (2009). Social support as a mediator of psychological distress in firefighters. *The Irish Journal of Psychology, 30*(1-2), 87-98. doi:10.1080/03033910.2009.10446300.

Regehr, C., Hill, J., Knott, T., and Sault, B. (2003). Social support, self-efficacy and trauma in new recruits and experienced firefighters. *Stress and Health, 19*(4), 189-193.

Reivich, K. and Shatté, A. (2002). *The resilience factor: 7 Essential skills for overcoming life's inevitable obstacles.* New York, NY: Broadway Books.

Rutter, M. (1987). Psychosocial resilience and protective mechanisms. *American Journal of Orthopsychiatry, 57*(3), 316-331.

Ryan, R. M. and Deci, E. L. (2000). Self-determination theory and the facilitation of intrinsic motivation, social development, and well-being. *American Psychologist, 55*(1), 68-78.

Shakespeare-Finch, J., Rees, A., and Armstrong, D. (2014). Social support, self-efficacy, trauma and well-being in emergency medical dispatchers. *Social Indicators Research*, 1-17.

Sherman, D. K., Bunyan, D. P., Creswell, J. D., and Jaremka, L. M. (2009). Psychological vulnerability and stress: the effects of self-affirmation on sympathetic nervous system responses to naturalistic stressors. *Health Psychology, 28*(5), 554-562.

Sonnentag, S., and Grant, A. M. (2012). Doing good at work feels good at home, but not right away: When and why perceived prosocial impact predicts positive affect. *Personnel Psychology, 65*(3), 495-530.

Taylor, S. E. (2010). Mechanisms linking early life stress to adult health outcomes. *Proceedings of the National Academy of Sciences, 107*(19), 8507-8512.

Van Orden, K. A., Witte, T. K., Cukrowicz, K. C., Braithwaite, S. R., Selby, E. A., and Joiner Jr, T. E. (2010). The interpersonal theory of suicide. *Psychological Review, 117*(2), 575-600.

Varvel, S. J., He, Y., Shannon, J. K., Tager, D., Bledman, R. A., Chaichanasakul, A., Mendoza, M. M., and Mallinckrodt, B. (2007). Multidimensional, threshold effects of social support in firefighters: Is more support invariably better? *Journal of Counseling Psychology, 54*(4), 458-465.

Chapter 6
Discussion

The research described in this paper points toward three major factors that influence the degree to which firefighter emergency responders exhibit resilience in the face of adverse events. These factors, when they are present, have the potential to prevent or mitigate psychological distress following stressful or traumatic situations. When these factors are absent, they can lead to or exacerbate such distress. To recap:

- **Realistic optimistic thinking**. This type of thinking is what often results when a person makes a habit of thinking flexibly, accurately, and thoroughly (Reivich 2015). It includes positive appraisals of one's influence and effectiveness on the job and perceived prosocial impact, or the belief that one's efforts are helpful to others. Negative self-appraisals, which are associated with psychological distress, are evidence of inaccurate, pessimistic thinking patterns. Realistic thinking does not have to equate with negative thinking patterns. Even if more accurate thinking leads to the conclusion that someone is partly or fully responsible for a problem, it puts that person in a better mindset to seek solutions (Gillham et al. 2014).
- **Social support**. In particular, perceived social support, or knowing that support is available if needed, tends to be more beneficial than received support (Prati and Pietrantoni 2010). Support from supervisors is particularly important (Varvel et al. 2007). There is some indication that the amount of social support decreases later in a firefighter's career (Chamberlin and Green 2010; Regehr et al. 2003). Additionally, decreasing negative social interactions may be just as important as increasing social support (Farnsworth and Sewell 2011).
- **Self-efficacy for coping**. A firefighter's belief that he or she can take action to deal effectively with a stressful event is associated with less psychological distress and better event outcomes. Additionally, the level of perceived coping self-efficacy can predict whether social support and optimism will result in a resilient response to traumatic events (e.g., Benight and Bandura 2004).

As the research indicates, these three factors are not isolated. Rather, they are interrelated in their effects. Prolonged distress in response to trauma is often accompanied by more than one of these factors, if not all three in combination. All three factors are often cited in studies that examine the coping measures used by firefighters to facilitate more adaptive responses in stressful situations. For example, in a study of emergency workers including firefighters mentioned in Chap. 5 (McCammon et al. 1988), workers were asked to cite effective coping strategies. Those strategies involved reframing how they think about the situation to make it more tolerable. Reframing comprised feeling a sense of mastery or self-efficacy about the situation; developing positive appraisals about their role in the incident; and generally looking at the situation in adaptive ways that facilitate coping. Facilitators of recovery from trauma among the emergency workers included a commitment to their profession, the cohesiveness of workers in the organization, and the satisfaction they experienced from helping others (McCammon et al. 1988).

Thus, it is necessary to consider all three factors—realistic optimistic thinking, perceived social support, and perceived self-efficacy for coping—in order to effectively promote resilient responses in the firefighter emergency responder population. Together, they are considered a set of potent psychosocial resources that can protect against the psychological and physiological harm caused by stress (Taylor 2010).

The literature reviewed in this paper provides indications that realistic optimistic thinking, as well as real and perceived social support, lead to greater perceptions of self-efficacy for coping with stressful situations. For example, many of the studies cited in this paper link negative, unrealistic, and out-of-perspective thinking patterns with low self-efficacy for coping (e.g., Bryant and Guthrie 2007; McCammon et al. 1988; Milen 2009; Van Orden et al. 2010). At the same time, less psychological distress is associated with more optimistic but realistic thinking that results in increased feelings of satisfaction, positive emotion, and competence for the job (e.g., McCammon et al. 1988; Sonnentag and Grant 2012). In addition, optimistic thinking is associated with a greater tendency to seek solutions to problems, which is an active coping strategy (Gillham et al. 2014). Perceived self-efficacy is predicated on having the belief and confidence that one can handle challenging situations and shape their outcome (Benight and Bandura 2004).

From the perspective of Self-Determination Theory, research indicates that a supportive social environment helps to provide motivation to develop mastery over one's environment (Ryan and Deci 2000). Lower levels of perceived social support were also associated with lower levels of self-efficacy and increased psychological distress in experienced firefighters (Regehr et al. 2003). Finally, the research by Benight and Bandura (2004) points out that social support and optimism both lead to and account for the increase in coping self-efficacy that minimizes psychological distress in the face of the resource loss caused by traumatic situations.

Based on this research, the interventions summarized below for increasing social support and developing skills for realistic optimistic thinking—assuming they are practiced enough to the point of being automatic and habitual—are predicted to lead to the perceived coping self-efficacy that is so important to resilience. Further, measured increases in coping self-efficacy could serve as a marker for whether interventions to increase social support and optimistic thinking are having their desired effects.

But beyond increases in coping self-efficacy that might be predicted through increases in realistic optimistic thinking and social support, research indicates that it is possible to successfully apply specific interventions to increase coping self-efficacy directly. This can be done in a number of ways. It can be done by changing one's mindset about stress from negative (stress is a threat) to positive (stress is a challenge) (Jamieson et al. 2013) and by choosing to see stress as a state that enhances, rather than hinders, performance (Crum et al. 2013). It can be done by transforming stressful experiences into meaningful experiences that help us to reinforce and affirm our values (Cohen and Sherman 2014). It can also be done by connecting the stressful experience to a larger life purpose (McGonigal 2015).

6.1 Sample Interventions

All three of these factors—realistic optimistic thinking; social support; and coping self-efficacy—can be addressed in the context of a primary prevention program of interventions to increase resilient thinking, emotions, and behaviors in firefighter emergency responders. The objectives would be to first, prepare first responders psychologically so that extreme adverse reactions to traumatic events are prevented or mitigated, and second, to help emergency responders deal more productively and effectively with the everyday stresses that occur at work, at home, and in life. Accumulated stresses, over time, can take their toll on a responder's ability to be resilient in a given situation.

This proposed approach is intended to supplement, not replace, the programs that are already in place or being developed for the fire service that address secondary and tertiary prevention needs. Programs that attempt to reduce the impact of a traumatic event that has already occurred, or to mitigate the long-term effects of an adverse reaction to a traumatic event, are needed every bit as much as fire suppression is needed alongside fire prevention efforts.

The research advises that the most effective approach to resilience training is to apply interventions at three levels: the level of the individual, the level of relationships (both work-related and personal), and the level of the environment or organization (Luthar and Cicchetti 2000). Firefighter emergency responder resilience training should be incorporated into all three levels, each reinforcing the other.

The interventions summarized in this chapter are based on factors identified in the literature review as being associated with increased resilience and reduced psychological distress in relation to trauma. In this case, they would be introduced as a primary prevention measure and take place before the traumatic event occurs. The goal is to teach a set of tools for developing mental toughness. That includes preventing and mitigating the symptoms of traumatic stress, as well as enabling more adaptive responses to adverse events generally. For each intervention, specific examples would be developed that are tailored to real-life situations encountered by firefighter emergency responders. The more they are practiced, the more habitual and automatic they will become. Some of the interventions are described in more detail in the Supplement at the end of this chapter.

6.1.1 Interventions to Increase Realistic Optimistic Thinking

- **Identifying ABCs: A foundational skill to build resilience**. This intervention is based on a model developed by psychologist Albert Ellis, a pioneer in the field of cognitive behavioral therapies, to identify common thought patterns that can either provide helpful or counterproductive responses to events (Ellis 2003; Reivich and Shatté 2002). The intervention teaches how to identify beliefs (B), defined as heat-of-the-moment thoughts that are triggered by activating events (A). Activating events are simply what happened. The beliefs result in emotions, behaviors, bodily reactions and other responses that in this model are called consequences (C). In most cases, at least one belief connects an activating event and a consequence. Evaluating the B-C connections can help us to see if we tend to respond in one particular style more than others. This intervention is included in the U.S. Army's Master Resilience Training (MRT) as part of the "Building Mental Toughness" module (Reivich et al. 2011).
- **Identifying thinking traps and getting FAT thinking**. This is another lesson taught as part of the MRT's "Building Mental Toughness" module (Reivich et al. 2011). Building on the ABC model, this lesson teaches how to identify thinking traps. Thinking traps are destructive thinking patterns that cause us to miss critical information and lead us to draw inaccurate conclusions about situations. Thinking traps interfere with resilience because they make us less able to assess the facts, and less able to respond appropriately to the situation (Reivich and Shatté 2002). But if we can recognize when we are in danger of falling into a thinking trap, we can learn to ask critical questions that lead to Flexible, Accurate, and Thorough (FAT) thinking (Reivich 2015).
- **Counteracting unproductive thoughts in real time**. Another of the MRT lessons involves changing counterproductive beliefs at the time that they occur, so that, over time, fewer such thoughts occur and when they do, they are less destructive (Reivich and Shatté 2002). The skill involves applying one of three strategies to the negative thought in the moment and reframing it to be more productive, as in Table 6.1.
- **Hunting the good stuff**. This exercise involves either individually or in a group reflecting on ways that the firefighters and/or their shift helped others or otherwise made the world a better place, and what each positive experience or event meant to them individually. It is intended to enhance positive emotions and develop feelings of perceived prosocial impact at the end of the day or at the

Table 6.1 Counteracting unproductive thoughts in real time (Reivich et al. 2011; Reivich and Shatté 2002)

Strategy	What you say to yourself
Optimism	A more accurate way to look at this is…
Evidence	That's not true because…
Perspective	A more likely outcome is… and I can … to deal with it

end of a shift. Hunting the Good Stuff is based on an intervention called Three Good Things, which was shown to increase happiness and decrease depressive symptoms for six months after it was practiced for a week by participants recruited from the authentichappiness.org website (Seligman et al. 2005). This activity is similar to an exercise taught during the MRT (Reivich et al. 2011). It is intended to supplement the after-action reviews that take place routinely in fire departments, which focus on how to improve operations.

6.1.2 Interventions to Increase the Quality of Social Interactions

- **Active-constructive responding**. How someone responds to the good news shared by another matters. Of four main styles of responding, only *one* has been shown to have positive implications for the relationship: Active-Constructive Responding (ACR). ACR involves showing authentic support and asking good questions, as opposed to a positive but passive response (passive-constructive), an engaged but deflating response (active-destructive), or ignoring the news altogether (passive-destructive) (Gable et al. 2004). People who respond actively and constructively to others' good news report greater relationship satisfaction, higher quality relationships, and fewer conflicts (Lambert et al. 2012a, b). This intervention is used as part of the Strengthening Relationships module of the MRT for building relationships with other soldiers and with their family members (Reivich et al. 2011).
- **Building high-quality connections**. High-quality connections (HQCs) are short-term positive interactions at work between two people. This training might take the format of a workshop with follow-up. All department members would be trained first on what HQCs are and the various benefits that have been documented in interpersonal and organizational contacts. Second, they would learn the mechanisms by which HQCs can be achieved (emotional, cognitive, and behavioral). Third, they would learn the pathways within each mechanism, which provide specific techniques for achieving HQCs (Stephens et al. 2011). Department members would then be asked to consciously foster HQCs within the fire department. Members would then be responsible for reporting on at least 3 HQCs they achieved every day that they are working at the department. Department members also would be encouraged to create HQCs outside work.

6.1.3 Interventions to Increase Coping Self-efficacy

- **Reappraising your stress response**. This intervention involves the facilitator sharing research results that show that the physical ways that the body reacts to stress actually can result in positive outcomes. They help to focus attention, increase motivation and otherwise help one rise to the challenge. They help one to be more prosocial, experience less fear and more courage, and otherwise strengthen social ties. They also contribute to mental processes that help us learn and grow from stressful experiences (e.g., Jamieson et al. 2013). The facilitator then asks participants to reflect on a recent stressful experience in their own life, and choose to rethink the stress response as evidence that their bodies and brains were helping them to cope. Participants next write about their experience from the reappraised viewpoint, and consider how they might use their personal resources to turn a future stressful situation from a threat to a challenge (McGonigal 2015).
- **Tying stressful situations to meaning, values, and larger-than-self goals**. A facilitator shares research about prosocial behavior and its benefits. These benefits include helpful effects on the body's response to stress, the importance of prosocial impact to a meaningful life, and the ways in which reflecting on personal values leads to more approach-oriented ways of dealing with stress (e.g., Cohen and Sherman 2014; Grant and Sonnentag 2010; Poulin and Holman 2013). The facilitator leads a discussion about identifying one's most important personal values, and how those values reflect the choices and goals one makes in life. The facilitator asks participants to reflect in writing and then in follow-up discussion about how a situation in their life that causes them to feel stress is important, and why. Reasons could include that the stressful situation expresses and honors their values, gives their life greater meaning, and/or helps them to achieve goals that go beyond satisfying personal needs (larger-than-self goals). The facilitator encourages participants to practice reminding themselves in the future of how a stressful situation on the job, at home, or in other important areas of their life is helping to serve a larger purpose. This would be a particularly challenging exercise in light of situations that are not easily seen as serving a larger purpose (such as an ugly divorce, or a particularly tragic and horrific incident that was preventable). Practice will help improve the coping response, and it will become easier to see that how one responds to stress is a choice (McGonigal 2015).

6.1.4 Measurement Tools

Measuring the effectiveness of any applied interventions that are part of a firefighter resilience training program is vital. This is in keeping with positive psychology's emphasis on measurement and science-based interventions, as well as the fire

6.1 Sample Interventions   57

service's own call for "evidence-supported practices and techniques" to address behavioral health (National Fallen Firefighters Foundation 2011, p. 34). Program measurement helps the fire service justify interventions that demonstrate a positive difference. Specific measures would be explored and determined during development and pilot testing of the training program. However, this section discusses some criteria for consideration.

Existing instruments are preferable to creating new scales from scratch, as long as they measure the variables that the training program hopes to influence. Existing measures are also likely to have undergone testing for reliability and validity. Reliability refers to whether the assessment produces similar results under consistent conditions. Validity is the degree to which the assessment measures what it intends to measure, and whether it can be used with audiences beyond that for which it was originally developed. A new test should be considered only if existing tests cannot be found that appropriately apply, or can be modified to apply, to the emergency responder audience.

Fire departments have limited time and resources to devote to any single training effort. Shorter measures, and those that are easy to score and interpret, are preferable, particularly if a combination of measures is to be used. Given the variety of factors the proposed resilience training intends to influence, a single measure is not likely to capture them all effectively.

Ideally, some consensus on the measures used would help to compare results from department to department. A schedule would need to be developed for administering the tests before and after training, with proper controls. Long-term follow-up should be considered in light of studies that show that the effects of resilience interventions increase over time (e.g., Cutuli et al. 2013). In addition, self-report measures could be supplemented by direct-observation reporting by the department chief and by shift officers prior to the intervention and periodically thereafter that look at factors such as absenteeism, prosocial behavior on the job, and the quality of social interactions. The combination of self-report and third-party reports can add to the validity of the results.

Some instruments to consider, based on the areas the resilience training intends to improve:

- Two instruments are appropriate for measuring the impact of interventions to foster realistic optimistic thinking, which correlates with a greater tendency to problem solve (Gillham et al. 2014). One is the Life Orientation Test—Revised (LOT-R), a 10-item self-report measure that was developed to assess individual differences in optimism and pessimism (Carver et al. 2010). The other, which measures short-term moods, is the Positive and Negative Affect Schedule (PANAS), a 10-item self-report measure that assesses positive and negative emotions on separate scales (Watson et al. 1988).
- The Professional Quality of Life: Compassion Satisfaction and Fatigue Version 5 (ProQOL) is appropriate for measuring interventions intended to influence positive emotion and perceived prosocial impact. The ProQOL is a 30-item

self-report measure that assesses how one feels in relation to both the positive and negative aspects of one's work in the helping professions (Hudnall Stamm 2009).
- Two measures are appropriate to assess interventions intended to lead to stronger interpersonal relationships and greater social support. One is an adaptation of the Sources of Social Support Scale (SSSS), a self-report measure that assesses the kinds of help and support obtained from key individuals in the respondent's life (Carver 2006). The other is a 10-item self-report questionnaire on High Quality Connections (HQC) developed and validated by Carmeli and Gittell (2009). The HQC questionnaire rates the extent to which the respondent experiences three features of high quality relationships—shared goals, shared knowledge, and mutual respect—at the organizational level.
- Three instruments to measure changes in coping self-efficacy include the Firefighter Coping Self-Efficacy Scale (Lambert et al. 2012a, b), the Revised Ways of Coping Checklist for Firefighters (Dowdall-Thomae et al. 2012), and the Brief COPE (Carver 1997).
- The 8-item Stress Mindset Measure (Crum et al. 2013) can gauge whether interventions intended to change one's relationship to stress are having an effect. Fire department leaders and supervisors, however, would be more interested in observable behavioral indicators of reduced stress. Performance indicators include improved decision making, better time management, decreases in absenteeism and presenteeism (coming into work while sick), and less tardiness. Social indicators include fewer withdrawal behaviors and better social interactions on the job.

The instruments described above are individual measures. Assessments pertaining to aspects of department-wide effectiveness would require further discussion.

6.2 The Case for Universal Training

Resilience training potentially benefits *all* firefighters. It should be applied universally to all members of a department rather than just to those who are identified as being "at risk" for psychological distress. Training on the physical aspects of firefighting proceeds on the basis that the more it is practiced, the more it becomes part of muscle memory. Thus, the correct actions are carried out automatically when the need arises. Making resilience skills a habit will lead to their being part of the "mental muscle memory" automatically applied when faced with challenging situations. These skills then become an ingrained manner of coping. Moreover, an intervention that is framed as "training" is more likely to be accepted than if it were presented as "treatment." Treatment implies that the recipients need help and imparts a stigma on the situation.

Because there is no way of accurately predicting who will have a house fire in the future, we prudently teach fire prevention to everyone. In a similar way, we do not necessarily know which firefighters will benefit most from resilience training. However, the skills and techniques of training can be applied not only in the case of traumatic events but also to everyday stresses. Resilience is exhibited on a situation-specific basis (Rutter 1987). Someone who has demonstrated resilience in the past may be unexpectedly challenged by a "perfect storm" of circumstances in the future that has the potential to overwhelm coping strategies that worked well before.

As a matter of fairness, all firefighters should have the exposure to resilience training and the opportunity to apply it in all areas of their lives, both on and off duty. Additionally, if all firefighters were to receive the same or similar training, they would have a common language and frame of reference with which to discuss and practice coping strategies, and to reinforce those skills in one another.

6.2.1 Implementation and Cultural Considerations

Incorporating resilience training skills into firefighter recruit school would be an excellent opportunity to introduce resilience training skills to a large group of firefighters at the beginning of their careers. As those new to the fire service learn the basics of being a firefighter emergency responder, resilience training could potentially have the greatest impact. However, while the training should be introduced in recruit school, it by no means should end there. Research demonstrates that resilience and coping self-efficacy are not considered stable personality traits but rather are dependent on the situation and environment (Lambert et al. 2012a, b). In addition, research indicates that social support can wane over the course of firefighter careers (Regehr et al. 2003). Thus, resilience skills should be taught early and reinforced often. Fellow fire service members as training facilitators may be the best approach. Some studies report that firefighters can be uncomfortable receiving training from those who do not have direct experience as first responders themselves. They believe that outsiders cannot relate to the traumatic experiences first responders encounter (Jahnke et al. 2014).

A practical way to incorporate resilience training into a fire department's routine is through existing peer support providers. Peer support is already a recommended component of fire service behavioral health programs (Wilmoth 2014). Expanding the role of peer support providers to practice resilience interventions from a primary prevention perspective enhances the function they serve in assisting firefighters in psychological distress.

Ideally, the fire department should be where resilience skills get reinforced. That entails a "train-the-trainer" training for key individuals within the department on how to use the skills. These individuals in turn would train others within the department to use them, along the model employed by the U.S. Army's Master Resilience Training (Reivich et al. 2011). Shift or company officers, responsible for a team of first responders within the fire department, are a logical group to receive the initial training. They play a key role as both formal and informal leaders within the department.

Retired fire department members may be another natural avenue for providing resilience training. Retirees are at increased risk for suicide due to a loss of identity, purpose, and social support that they had as a member of the fire department. This is particularly true early in retirement (IAFF Behavioral Wellness Manual n.d.; Sivak 2016). Equipping retired department members to assist in providing resilience training to active members and to help reinforce that training within the department on a regular basis is an excellent use of an under-used resource. Additionally, it would provide retirees with a responsibility that would add identity, meaning, social contact, and increased well-being to their own lives. Training retirees to be resilience trainers would, incidentally, supply the retirees themselves with useful coping skills.

Finally, veterans who have been exposed to the U.S. Army's resilience training and subsequently join or return to their fire departments back home would have an excellent background with which to teach resilience skills to their fellow department members and help to reinforce those skills among their peers as they become habits.

6.2.2 Moving Toward a More Resilient Fire Service

Training is a big part of a firefighter's life. After the initial training to get basic certification as a firefighter (some 600 h over the course of approximately 12 weeks or more), there are other requirements. These include training based on keeping one's basic certification, advancing to new levels of expertise and responsibility within the department, developing knowledge and skills for special operations and situations, separate training for emergency medical response, and required annual continuing education depending on the jurisdiction. Each shift in a department spends considerable time training and drilling to keep their skills sharp when they are not responding to calls. So, how will another training program go over when firefighters already spend so much of their time training?

As firefighters well know, training is how people get good at things. Training and drilling enables not only the muscle memory to perform a task correctly each time, but it also helps to develop the confidence—indeed, the *self-efficacy*—of knowing that he or she can handle the situation when it occurs in real life. Training on the physical aspects of the firefighter's job is a given. Training on the psychological aspects to develop the coping self-efficacy for weathering stressful events is arguably just as important, but traditionally is not given the attention it deserves.

At the same time, fire departments likely will not have the luxury of a concentrated 10-day training such as the one provided through the U.S. Army's Master Resilience Training. However, a smaller package of interventions administered over a more manageable time frame can also be effective. The U.S. Navy's

BOOT STRAP training comprised one weekly 45 min session over a 9-week period (Williams et al. 2004). Other research has supported the effectiveness of brief interventions to change mindsets and behaviors in a lasting way (Dweck 2008; Crum et al. 2013; Cohen and Sherman 2014). Most of the interventions recommended in this Brief can be delivered in short sessions of one hour or less. The key is the extent to which they are practiced and reinforced over time. As data on their effectiveness accumulates, interventions can be refined and added.

Having the buy-in of fire chiefs and training directors is absolutely crucial to initiating a resilience training program. Progressive chiefs are needed to agree to pilot the approach in their departments, as well as chiefs who are willing to have their departments serve as controls. Next steps include refining the elements of the training and collecting evidence that shows it is effective for the fire service population.

Beyond helping to define and refine the training, chiefs are also needed to help define the organizational aspect of this effort. What does a resilient fire department look like? What conditions in a department lead to an environment that encourages resilience in its members? How do its members contribute to a stronger and more efficient operation? What values, leadership, policies, guidelines, practices, energies, relationships, and systems must be in place to create an environment that makes resilience possible? Research suggests departments can build resilience in their members by fostering realistic optimistic thinking; stronger social support networks; and greater levels of individual and collective coping self-efficacy. How can we measure these effects to determine if and how they can lead to a more efficient and effective fire department and fire service as a whole? The work to identify, define and measure the mechanisms and effects of resilient fire departments is a study waiting to be conducted.

6.3 Limitations of This Review

When considering the factors related to psychological distress in firefighter emergency responders, many of the studies cited here were limited to that population. Relying too heavily on research results that did not include the firefighter emergency responder population prompts questions about whether the conclusions are applicable to the population of interest. At the same time, not all of the studies looking at firefighter emergency responder populations took place in the United States, so questions might be raised about whether the same population in different countries are comparable in terms of types of experiences, reactions to traumatic events, and response to interventions.

Studies cited in this Brief often used different measures to assess constructs such as the impact of traumatic events, self-efficacy, and sources of support. It simply was not practical to reference only studies that used identical measures. While that variation introduces some question of whether the measures were in fact assessing exactly the same concepts, the manifestations of similar constructs often overlap and interrelate despite nuanced differences in how they are defined. For example, self-efficacy, mastery, agency, and competence describe related concepts. Thus, the authors treated similar concepts as falling under the same umbrella construct in order to make useful connections.

Most of the studies referred to in this Brief used self-report measures. While being the most widely used type of measurement, self-report measures can have limitations. They are subject to sources of error such as faking, situational influences (for example, a rainy day might affect a response), social desirability bias (responding based on what the respondent thinks the researcher wants to see), and response sets (following an arbitrary rule such as responding with the same answer to all questions regardless of what is true) (A. Duckworth personal communication September 3, 2014). In some of the studies cited, self-report measures are supplemented by informant (third-party) reports or other more objective and independent measures, which add to the validity of the results. Still, the results from each study tend to be consistent with one another, which suggests that any variation introduced by self-report measures did not change the overall conclusions of this paper.

Studies of resilience training programs on school-age children and military populations present suggestions for interventions that could work with a firefighter emergency responder population, but they are just suggestions until they can be tried and tested with this population.

6.4 Future Directions

This Brief is just the beginning of an inquiry into how positive psychology concepts, science, and interventions can be applied to improve the resilience of the men and women who make up the fire and emergency services. Through the strengthening of realistic optimistic thinking, greater social support, and improved self-efficacy for coping with challenging circumstances, the goal of this effort is to enhance emergency responders' ability to withstand traumatic stresses, and improve their overall psychological functioning in the course of their everyday activities both on and off the job.

A study based on this research would assemble and pilot-test a package of interventions within a number of fire departments in various geographical regions and makeups (career, volunteer, combination) in a "train-the-trainer" model such as that used for the Army's Master Resilience Training. Because the results of such training may take time to become apparent in terms of preventing or mitigating PTSD, depression, and other symptoms of psychological distress, interim measures of effectiveness may need to be put in place.

The positive psychology sub-field of positive organizational scholarship (POS) has much to teach us about creating an environment that fosters resilience. The POS literature would inform a study to determine which factors and characteristics contribute to resilient fire departments in terms of leadership, values, practices, policies, and membership. A study looking at resilience at the fire department level and testing interventions to create such environments is absolutely crucial to ensuring that a program of resilience training will "stick," because the most effective interventions take into account the individual, relationship, and environmental levels in a multi-faceted approach (Luthar and Cicchetti 2000).

Future research should look at interventions that foster realistic optimistic thinking, stronger social support, coping self-efficacy, and other relevant constructs in populations besides those in the education and the military examples. Studies of resilience training in high-performance professions such as elite athletes and athletic teams are an example of another possible avenue of inquiry that could be applicable to firefighter emergency responders.

Also, the study of strengths-based resilience, in which character strengths are incorporated into efforts to enhance protective factors that promote resilience, was not examined in this paper. However, strengths-based resilience offers a fertile area of exploration that would no doubt complement the approaches suggested here. Identifying and using one's signature strengths in new ways, for example, could provide opportunities to practice mastery and enhance feelings of self-efficacy.

It is reasonable to believe that the benefits of resilience training will not be limited to preventing psychological distress reactions to trauma but also to fostering better cohesion, teamwork, and retention within the fire department. Based on what we know about organization-wide benefits of military applications of resilience training (Williams et al. 2007; Harms et al. 2013), this appears to be a promising area of future study.

6.5 Supplement

What could fire department resilience training consist of? What might it look like? One approach is to choose interventions that have been tested in other domains and tailor them to the fire service audience. Presented here are four examples of interventions that target the factors identified as critical to developing flexible, accurate, thorough thinking, and developing positive emotions through realistic optimism. These techniques are based on interventions taught as part of the Master Resilience Training in the U.S. Army (Reivich et al. 2011).

Next are two interventions that target factors demonstrated to lead to stronger relationships both at work and in other areas of life. The Active-Constructive Responding intervention is based on a technique taught as part of the Master Resilience Training in the U.S. Army (Reivich et al. 2011). The Building High-Quality Connections intervention derives from research presented by the University of Michigan's Ross School of Business (Dutton 2003; Stephens et al. 2011).

6.5.1 Identifying ABCs—A Foundational Skill to Build Resilience

Background. If we can learn to identify the beliefs and thoughts that underlie our responses to events in our lives, we can be flexible in how we respond rather than falling back on a particular response or interpretive style every time. The ability to accurately assess a situation can allow us to evaluate whether our beliefs are contributing to making the situation better, or causing problems (Helping or Harming). The ABC model was developed by psychologist Albert Ellis, a pioneer in the field of cognitive behavioral therapies, as a tool to identify the beliefs that we have in response to events that lead to our emotions and behaviors (Ellis 2003; Reivich and Shatté 2002).

- The "A" stands for Activating Event: a "trigger" situation that can be big or small, resulting in beliefs that drive us to feel or act a certain way.
- The "B" stands for Beliefs. These are the "heat of the moment" thoughts, opinions, interpretations, and assumptions about what caused the Activating Event and what the implications might be. There are generally two types of beliefs that we are interested in: "Why" beliefs and "What Next" beliefs. There is usually at least one belief that connects an Activating Event and a Consequence.
- The "C" stands for Consequence. This is an emotion, behavior, physiological reaction or other result that stems from the Belief that we have about the Activating Event.

Once we identify the ABC, we can look for patterns in the B-C connection that indicates what our style of responding might be. For example, a common negative thought pattern is a belief that one has been harmed or violated in some way, with the corresponding consequences being anger and retaliation (Reivich and Shatté 2002). A common positive thought pattern is appreciation for what one has received, with associated consequences being gratitude and paying the favor back or forward (Fredrickson 2013). We can then evaluate each response pattern in terms of whether it helps or harms our ability to deal effectively with the Activating Event. The ABC technique can be used before, during, or after an Activating Event.

Implementation Steps: The facilitator presents the background. Group members provide examples of Activating Events and the facilitator leads the group to identify associated Beliefs and Consequences. The facilitator then reviews common patterns of B-C connections for both positive and negative Activating Events. Group members pair off to practice. Then the group reconvenes and the facilitator leads a discussion in which group members volunteer additional examples and raise questions that arose during the practice session.

6.5.2 Identifying Thinking Traps and Getting FAT Thinking

Background. This session begins with a review of the previous intervention on identifying the ABCs, then goes on to define Thinking Traps.

- **Remember the ABCs**. We all need to use shortcuts in our thinking to make sense of the world so that we are not assessing every situation as if we were encountering it for the first time. The fire service is familiar with using heuristic thinking and decision making, especially in emergencies, when time-critical decisions are made with limited information. However, sometimes in response to an (A) Activating Event, we get into destructive patterns of thinking, or (B) Beliefs, that cause us to miss critical information and lead us to draw inaccurate conclusions about situations, leading to harmful (C) Consequences (Ellis 2003). Those destructive patterns are known as Thinking Traps.
- **How Thinking Traps Interfere with Resilience**. We tend to fall into Thinking Traps when there is ambiguity about a situation; when we are tired, rundown, or stressed; and when we interact with those we are closest to. Because they cause us to miss information and respond in an overly rigid fashion, Thinking Traps make us less able to assess the facts, and less able to respond appropriately to the situation (Reivich and Shatté 2002).
- **Fixing the Problem: Get FAT**. The good news is that we can change our style of thinking if we do the hard work to understand the goals and ask critical questions that lead to FAT thinking: Flexible, Accurate, and Thorough (Reivich 2015). Participants may come to the conclusion that their initial belief was accurate, but most often the question will lead to a more even-handed way of looking at the situation.

For example, Personalizing is a common Thinking Trap, in which you attach all the responsibility and blame to yourself for what went wrong, failing to recognize the role that others played. To avoid the Personalizing Thinking Trap, look outward and ask how other people or the circumstances themselves contributed to the situation. Another common Thinking Trap is Tunnel Vision, focusing on insignificant details of the situation and missing the big picture. To avoid the Tunnel Vision Thinking Trap, broaden your view of the situation and ask what important information you missed the first time around (Reivich and Shatté 2002).

Implementation Steps: The facilitator provides background and reviews a list of the most common Thinking Traps, along with corresponding goals and critical questions for achieving more flexible, accurate, thorough thinking. The facilitator leads the group in some examples that might be encountered in the fire department. Group members pair off to practice, taking turns describing a situation from their lives (Activating Event) that prompted a destructive thinking pattern (Belief) and led to a harmful or negative result (Consequence). Partners can work together to determine the most likely Thinking Trap that was at work in the situation (Reivich and Shatté 2002). The group then reconvenes, and the facilitator leads a discussion at the end of the session in which participants volunteer examples as other group members contribute additional observations and suggestions, and raise questions.

6.5.3 Countering Unproductive Thoughts in Real Time

Background. Learning to counter unproductive thoughts and beliefs at the moment they occur is the essence of a skill called Real-time Resilience (Reivich and Shatté 2002). Excessive focus on inaccurately negative thoughts (or even unhelpful positive thoughts) can result in less confidence and engagement in performing tasks, which can put oneself and others at greater risk (Reivich et al. 2011). Once we develop the skill of recognizing our harmful beliefs and negative thoughts by way of the interventions described above, we can work on challenging them and reframing them to be more productive through our internal dialog. This is not a matter of automatically substituting positive thoughts for negative ones, but rather discovering the most accurate interpretation of events, which tends to result in more optimistic thinking.

With practice, the goal of Real-time Resilience is to have fewer nonproductive thoughts or less destructive thoughts when they do occur (Reivich and Shatté 2002). This will enable more of an ability and motivation to focus on completing the task at hand.

Implementation Steps. The facilitator reviews the background and presents examples for the group to work on together. They practice taking each example and applying the following three strategies to structure a response (Reivich and Shatté 2002):

- *Generate alternative beliefs: A more accurate way of seeing this is….* Think of a different and more accurate way to explain the situation than your heat-of-the-moment belief. Often, this will be a more optimistic and hopeful way of looking at the event.
- *Use evidence to test the accuracy of your beliefs: That's not true because….* Look for a specific and detailed example that challenges the unproductive belief.
- *Identify implications: A more likely outcome is….and I can….to deal with it.* To counter a tendency to think of the worst possible outcome of a situation, come up with a more realistic outcome and one thing that can be done to address it.

Group members briefly pair off to practice, and then reconvene for discussions and questions. The facilitator reviews common mistakes that are made with this exercise, and how to correct them (Reivich and Shatté 2002):

- *Using unrealistic optimism.* So-called Pollyanna optimism does not reflect the reality of the situation. If you remember that the goal is accuracy and not optimism, you will develop a sense of when your counter-thought is authentic to the situation rather than blindly idealistic.

- *Dismissing the grain of truth in the counter-productive beliefs.* If you automatically contradict the whole negative belief, you might miss the kernel of truth it holds, and it will not ring true. If you acknowledge the truth in the negative thought, you can identify a strategy to address it.
- *Blaming oneself or others.* Failure to acknowledge the proper responsibility of yourself or others in creating the situation denies you of the opportunity to take appropriate steps to address it. Often, both parties contribute to a problem. Try to minimize all-or-nothing thinking.
- *Minimizing the importance of the situation.* Denying the significance of the situation may result in substituting an unrealistic worst-case outcome with a similarly unrealistic best-case scenario. If the situation really does not matter, don't waste your energy on it. But if taking the most realistic view still acknowledges the problem, you will be in a better position to deal with it for having put it in perspective.

6.5.4 Hunting the Good Stuff

Background. As a way of enhancing positive emotions and developing feelings of perceived prosocial impact at the end of the day or at the end of a shift, this exercise involves either individually or in a group reflecting on ways that the firefighters and/or their shift helped others or otherwise made the world a better place, and what each positive experience or event meant to them. Similar to an exercise taught during the MRT (Reivich et al. 2011), Hunting the Good Stuff is based on an intervention called Three Good Things, which was shown to increase happiness and decrease depressive symptoms for six months after it was practiced for a week by participants recruited from the authentichappiness.org website (Seligman et al. 2005).

Reflecting on prosocial behavior has been found to be associated with positive emotion in firefighters that lasts even after the workday or shift is completed, and spills over into non-work environments (Sonnentag and Grant 2012). Focusing on the prosocial impacts of the job can help to make workers feel more competent and valued, as well as making them less likely to think negatively about themselves and their performance, and leading to less emotional exhaustion on the job (Grant and Sonnentag 2010).

This intervention is intended to supplement the after-action reviews that take place routinely in fire departments. Such reviews focus on how to prevent problems from happening again (which can, indeed, be a useful exercise and contribute to the safety climate of a department). But such reviews also focus on finding room to improve even when mistakes have not been made so that every incident becomes a learning experience. "Hunting the Good Stuff" is intended to build on the focus on the positive effects of the job, and to remind firefighters individually and collectively that their efforts are making a difference. Examples can be large or small.

They do not need to be big, momentous examples in order to be meaningful. Try to notice and appreciate small blessings, too.

Implementation Steps. The facilitator leads the group in answering the following questions in sequence.

- What happened today (or during this shift) that was good? (Come up with at least three examples individually or as a group.)
- (For each example) What did you (or your colleagues) do to contribute to the good event?
- What does the good thing mean to you (personally or as part of your group, department, or fire service)?
- What can you do to make this good event or something like it happen again in the future?

6.5.5 Active-Constructive Responding

Background. People benefit from sharing good news. When someone shares something positive with you, the technical term for this is *capitalization* (Langston 1994). There are potentially many opportunities to share positive information. Positive events occur at a 3:1 ratio to negative events, and people tend to share the best thing that happened that day 60–80 % of the time (Gable and Haidt 2005). Topics can range from routine events to more significant news. Capitalization has been shown to lead to increases in positive emotion, greater life satisfaction, and greater feelings of belonging. The more good news people share, the greater the benefits. (Lambert et al. 2012a, b).

The way you respond to the news of others matters! How you respond to someone's good news has implications for the person who shared and for the health of your relationship with that person. Of four main styles of responding, only *one* has been shown to have positive implications for the relationship: Active-Constructive Responding (ACR). The other styles of responding (even passive-constructive) have negative effects on relationships (Gable et al. 2004) (Table 6.2).

Benefits of Active-constructive Responding. Partners who give each other ACR report greater relationship satisfaction, greater intimacy (more understanding, caring, and trust) and a higher quality of relationship, with more daily happiness and fewer conflicts (Lambert et al. 2012a, b). Relationships are at a higher risk to break up if ACR is not present in the relationship (Gable et al. 2006).

Implementation Steps. The facilitator demonstrates each of the types of responding and discusses how they differ and how they make the recipient feel. Then the group practices ACR in one-on-one interactions, after which the facilitator leads a discussion and addresses questions. Discussion points might include how ACR can

Table 6.2 Only the active-constructive style of response has positive implications for relationships (Gable et al. 2004)

Style of response	Constructive	Destructive
Active	*Active-constructive*: Authentic support, ask positive questions	*Active-destructive*: Crush enthusiasm, raise negative issues
Passive	*Passive-constructive*: Subdued positive response, no follow-up	*Passive-destructive*: Ignore event, change subject

be done in an authentic way when the responder is not "feeling" it, and whether every piece of good news shared requires the same level of acknowledgement.

6.5.6 Building High-Quality Connections (HQCs)

Background. *What are High-Quality Connections and why do they matter?* HQCs are brief positive interactions between two people at work—either between strangers or within ongoing relationships (Stephens et al. 2011). Among other benefits, HQCs have been found to improve working memory, cardiovascular and immune functioning, and recovery and adaptation from loss or illness in both people involved in the interaction (Stephens et al. 2011). At the organizational level, HQCs are associated with higher levels of psychological safety, which can result in greater learning from failures; with higher levels of trust, which can lead to greater cooperation; and with improved coordination and detection of errors (Stephens et al. 2011).

How are HQCs formed? HQCs can develop through three mechanisms (Stephens et al. 2011). Cognitive, or mental, processes include awareness of what others are doing, impressions of warmth and accepting, and taking the perspective of others. Emotional processes include sharing positive emotions; mimicking another's positive facial expressions, movements, and vocalizations; and feeling empathy toward another person. Behavioral mechanisms include showing esteem, dignity, and caring for others through respectful engagement; helping others perform or complete a task through task enabling; and bonding outside the normal work roles and behaviors in a light-hearted way through play.

Implementation Steps. The plan is for the intervention to take place in 45 min sessions once a week for three weeks. During this time, all fire department members are trained and encouraged to develop and maintain HQCs with their fellow department members. The key objective would be to create a culture of HQCs that would lead to a more cohesive workplace that is better able to function on a day-to-day basis as well as to withstand the more stressful events that may occur long-term.

Week 1: All department members are trained on what high-quality connections are, the mechanisms by which they can be achieved (emotional, cognitive, and behavioral), and the pathways within each mechanism, which provide specific ways of achieving HQCs (Dutton 2003; Stephens et al. 2011).

All department members at the chief level (department chief, assistant chiefs, deputy chiefs, battalion chiefs) would receive an additional briefing during Week 1 on ways of establishing organizational values, policies, and practices within each of the mechanisms to foster HQCs around shared goals, shared knowledge, and mutual respect (Carmeli and Gittell 2009). With the help of a facilitator, they would decide which values, policies, and practices to put into place and inform their members.

Weeks 2 and 3: Department members are asked to consciously foster HQCs within the fire department and to be responsible for at least 3 HQCs every day that they are working at the department during those weeks. They will be given every-other-day email reminders and tips, as well as signs posted around the fire stations with suggestions for creating HQCs. Department members also would be encouraged to create HQCs outside work, but they would not be responsible for reporting on them. A check-in would take place between weeks 2 and 3 in order to informally gauge progress, answer questions and course-correct if necessary.

References

Benight, C. C., and Bandura, A. (2004). Social cognitive theory of posttraumatic recovery: The role of perceived self-efficacy. *Behaviour Research and Therapy, 42*(10), 1129-1148.

Bryant, R. A., and Guthrie, R. M. (2007). Maladaptive self-appraisals before trauma exposure predict posttraumatic stress disorder. *Journal of Consulting and Clinical Psychology, 75*(5), 812-815.

Carmeli, A., and Gittell, J. H. (2009). High-quality relationships, psychological safety, and learning from failures in work organizations. *Journal of Organizational Behavior, 30,* 709-729. doi:10.1002/job.565.

Carver, C. S. (1997). You want to measure coping but your protocol's too long: Consider the Brief COPE. *International Journal of Behavioral Medicine*, 4, 92-100.

Carver, C. S. (2006). Sources of Social Support Scale. http://www.psy.miami.edu/faculty/ccarver/sclSSSS.html. Accessed 27 Feb 2016.

Carver, C. S., Scheier, M. F., and Segerstrom, S. C. (2010). Optimism. *Clinical Psychology Review, 30,* 879-889.

Chamberlin, M. J. A., and Green, H. J. (2010). Stress and coping strategies among firefighters and recruits. *Journal of Loss and Trauma, 15*(6), 548-560. doi:10.1080/15325024.2010.519275.

Cohen, G. L., and Sherman, D. K. (2014). The psychology of change: Self-affirmation and social psychological intervention. *Annual Review of Psychology, 65,* 333-371.

Crum, A. J., Salovey, P., and Achor, S. (2013). Rethinking stress: The role of mindsets in determining the stress response. *Journal of Personality and Social Psychology, 104*(4), 716-732.

Cutuli, J. J., Gillham, J. E., Chaplin, T. M., Reivich, K. J., Seligman, M. E. P., Gallop, R. J., ... and Freres, D. R. (2013). Preventing adolescents' externalizing and internalizing symptoms:

Effects of the Penn Resiliency Program. *The International Journal of Emotional Education*, 5(2), 67-79.

Dowdall-Thomae, C., Gilkey, J., Larson, W., and Arend-Hicks, R. (2012). Elite firefighter/first responder mindsets and outcome coping efficacy. *International Journal of Emergency Mental Health*, 14(4), 269-281.

Dutton, J. E. (2003). *Energize your workplace: How to create and sustain high-quality connections at work*. San Francisco, CA: Jossey-Bass.

Dweck, C. S. (2008). Can personality be changed? The role of beliefs in personality and change. *Current Directions in Psychological Science*, 17(6), 391-394.

Ellis, A. (2003). Early theories and practices of rational emotive behavior therapy and how they have been augmented and revised during the last three decades. *Journal of Rational-Emotive and Cognitive-Behavior Therapy*, 21(3/4), 219-243.

Farnsworth, J. K., and Sewell, K. W. (2011). Fear of emotion as a moderator between PTSD and firefighter social interactions. *Journal of Traumatic Stress*, 24(4), 444-450.

Fredrickson, B. L. (2013). Positive emotions broaden and build. *Advances in experimental social psychology*, 47, 1-53.

Gable, S. L., and Haidt, J. (2005). What (and why) is positive psychology? *Review of General Psychology*, 9(2), 103-110.

Gable, S. L., Reis, H. T., Impett, E. A., and Asher, E. R. (2004). What do you do when things go right? The intrapersonal and interpersonal benefits of sharing positive events. *Journal of Personality and Social Psychology*, 87, 228 –245.

Gable, S. L., Gonzaga, G. C., & Strachman, A. (2006). Will you be there for me when things go right? Supportive responses to positive event disclosures. *Journal of Personality and Social Psychology*, 91, 904 –917.

Gillham, J. E., Abenavoli, R. M., Brunwasser, S. M., Linkins, M., Reivich, K. J., and Seligman, M. E. P. (2014). Resilience education. In S. A. David, I. Boniwell, and A. Conley Ayers (Eds.), *The Oxford handbook of happiness* (pp. 609-630). Oxford, UK: Oxford University Press.

Grant, A. M., and Sonnentag, S. (2010). Doing good buffers against feeling bad: Prosocial impact compensates for negative task and self-evaluations. *Organizational Behavior and Human Decision Processes*, 111(1), 13-22.

Harms, P. D., Herian, M. N., Krasikova, D. V., Vanhove, A., and Lester, P. B. (2013). *The comprehensive soldier and family fitness program evaluation report #4: Evaluation of resilience training and mental and behavioral health outcomes*. Monterey, CA: Office of the Deputy Under Secretary of the Army.

Hudnall Stamm, B. (2009). *Professional Quality of Life: Compassion Satisfaction and Fatigue Version 5 (ProQOL)*. /www.isu.edu/ ∼ bhstamm or www.proqol.org.

International Association of Fire Fighters, AFL-CIO-CLC (n.d.). *Behavioral health*. https://www.iaff.org/HS/wfiresource/BehavioralHealth/behavioralhealth.html. Accessed 27 Feb 2016.

Jahnke, S. A., Gist, R., Poston, W. S. C., and Haddock, C. K. (2014). Behavioral health interventions in the fire service: Stories from the firehouse. *Journal of Workplace Behavioral Health*, 29(2), 113-126.

Jamieson, J. P., Mendes, W. B., and Nock, M. K. (2013). Improving acute stress responses: The power of reappraisal. *Current Directions in Psychological Science*, 22(1), 51-56.

Lambert, J. E., Benight, C. C., Harrison, E., and Cieslak, R. (2012a). The Firefighter Coping Self-Efficacy Scale: Measure development and validation. *Anxiety, Stress and Coping*, 25(1), 79-91.

Lambert, N. M., Gwinn, A. M., Baumeister, R. F., Strachman, A., Washburn, I. J., Gable, S. L., and Fincham, F. D. (2012b). A boost of positive affect: The perks of sharing positive experiences. *Journal of Social and Personal Relationships*, 1-20. doi:10.1177/0265407512449400.

Langston, C. A. (1994). Capitalizing on and coping with daily-life events: Expressive responses to positive events. *Journal of Personality and Social Psychology*, 67, 1112-1125.

Luthar, S. S., and Cicchetti, D. (2000). The construct of resilience: Implications for interventions and social policies. *Development and Psychopathology, 12*, 857-885.

McCammon, S., Durham, T. W., Allison Jr, E. J., and Williamson, J. E. (1988). Emergency workers' cognitive appraisal and coping with traumatic events. *Journal of Traumatic Stress, 1*(3), 353-372.

McGonigal, K. (2015). *The upside of stress: Why stress is good for you, and how to get good at it.* New York, NY: Penguin Random House.

Milen, D. (2009). The ability of firefighting personnel to cope with stress. *Journal of Social Change, 3*(1), 38-56.

National Fallen Firefighters Foundation (2011). *Report of the 2nd National Fire Service Research Agenda Symposium, May 20-22, 2011, National Fire Academy.*

Poulin, M. J., and Holman, E. A. (2013). Helping hands, healthy body? Oxytocin receptor gene and prosocial behavior interact to buffer the association between stress and physical health. *Hormones and Behavior, 63*(3), 510-517.

Prati, G., and Pietrantoni, L. (2010). The relation of perceived and received social support to mental health among first responders: A meta-analytic review. *Journal of Community Psychology, 38*(3), 403-417.

Regehr, C., Hill, J., Knott, T., and Sault, B. (2003). Social support, self-efficacy and trauma in new recruits and experienced firefighters. *Stress and Health, 19*(4), 189-193.

Reivich, K. (2015). *Positive psychology and individuals* [PowerPoint slides], January 30, 2015. Philadelphia, PA: The Trustees of the University of Pennsylvania.

Reivich, K. and Shatté, A. (2002). *The resilience factor: 7 Essential skills for overcoming life's inevitable obstacles.* New York, NY: Broadway Books.

Reivich, K. J., Seligman, M. E. P., and McBride, S. (2011). Master resilience training in the U.S. Army. *American Psychologist, 66*(1), 25-34. doi:10.1037/a0021897.

Rutter, M. (1987). Psychosocial resilience and protective mechanisms. *American Journal of Orthopsychiatry, 57*(3), 316-331.

Ryan, R. M. and Deci, E. L. (2000). Self-determination theory and the facilitation of intrinsic motivation, social development, and well-being. *American Psychologist, 55*(1), 68-78.

Seligman, M. E., Steen, T. A., Park, N., and Peterson, C. (2005). Positive psychology progress: Empirical validation of interventions. *American Psychologist, 60*(5), 410-421.

Sivak, C. (2016). Why firefighters take their own lives. *Fire Chief Digital 2*(1), 4-6. http://online.fliphtml5.com/jncs/vsfx/#p=1. Accessed 27 Feb 2016.

Sonnentag, S., and Grant, A. M. (2012). Doing good at work feels good at home, but not right away: When and why perceived prosocial impact predicts positive affect. *Personnel Psychology, 65*(3), 495-530.

Stephens, J. P., Heaphy, E., and Dutton, J. (2011). High-quality connections. In K. Cameron and G. Spreitzer (Eds.), *Handbook of positive organizational scholarship* (pp. 385-399). New York: Oxford University Press.

Taylor, S. E. (2010). Mechanisms linking early life stress to adult health outcomes. *Proceedings of the National Academy of Sciences, 107*(19), 8507-8512.

Van Orden, K. A., Witte, T. K., Cukrowicz, K. C., Braithwaite, S. R., Selby, E. A., and Joiner Jr, T. E. (2010). The interpersonal theory of suicide. *Psychological Review, 117*(2), 575-600.

Varvel, S. J., He, Y., Shannon, J. K., Tager, D., Bledman, R. A., Chaichanasakul, A., Mendoza, M. M., and Mallinckrodt, B. (2007). Multidimensional, threshold effects of social support in firefighters: Is more support invariably better? *Journal of Counseling Psychology, 54*(4), 458-465.

Watson, D., Clark, L. A., and Tellegen, A. (1988). Development and validation of brief measures of positive and negative affect: The PANAS scales. *Journal of personality and social psychology, 54*(6), 1063-1070.

Williams, A., Hagerty, B. M., Yousha, S. M., Horrocks, J., Hoyle, K. S., and Liu, D. (2004). Psychosocial effects of the Boot Strap intervention in Navy recruits. *Military Medicine, 169*(10), 814-820.

Williams, A., Hagerty, B. M., Andrei, A. C., Yousha, S. M., Hirth, R. A., and Hoyle, K. S. (2007). STARS: Strategies to assist Navy recruits' success. *Military Medicine, 172*(9), 942-949.

Wilmoth, J. A. (2014, May-June). Trouble in mind. Special report: Firefighter behavioral health. *NFPA Journal*. Quincy, MA: National Fire Protection Association. Retrieved from http://www.nfpa.org/newsandpublications/nfpa-journal/2014/may-june-2014/features/special-report-firefighter-behavioral-health. Accessed 27 Feb 2016.

Chapter 7
Conclusion

When the alarm sounds, we count on our firefighter emergency responders to show up and to be strong, both physically and psychologically. We expect this during our own time of need, for the needs of our neighbors, and again for the needs of our community members. These men and women are dedicated and courageous. They chose this path for themselves, and they train hard for the privilege of serving. At the same time, they do not get to choose the severity of the incidents to which they respond. They live the philosophy of "Other people matter" (Peterson 2006, p. 249) every day that they serve. But they are also human. They deserve to have access to every tool we know of and every opportunity available to strengthen their personal, social, and environmental resources so that they can carry out that job to the best of their capability.

Creating a more resilient fire service will ultimately mean challenging the fire service culture to put behavioral health on a par with physical fitness. Creating a more resilient fire service is also consistent with the best tendencies and instincts of the fire service to take care of its own.

This is a critically important goal and fully deserving of the resources that will be required to make it happen. It is not just about preventing PTSD, depression, and other signs and effects of psychological distress, but about creating a reduced vulnerability to everyday stressors as well. It is not only about cultivating the capacity in individuals to be less likely to succumb to long-term impairment when faced with harrowing scenarios at an uncommon pace and intensity. Ultimately, it is also about creating a more efficient, effective, and cohesive fire service in the

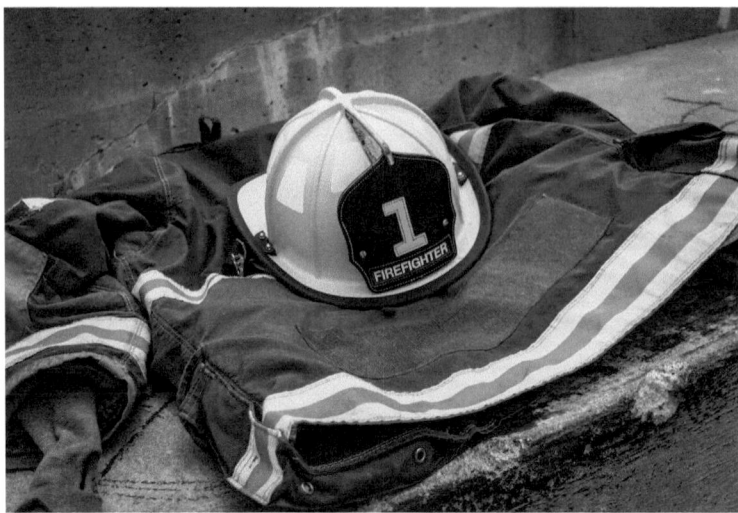

Fig. 7.1 Creative Commons Firefighter-920032 by The Hilary Clark, http://pixabay.com, licensed under CC0, public domain

process. In this most worthwhile pursuit, positive psychology may not have all the answers, but positive psychology can get us asking the right questions and headed in the right direction (Fig. 7.1).

Reference

Peterson, C. (2006). *A primer in positive psychology.* New York, NY: Oxford University Press.

Glossary of Terminology

Active-constructive responding A style of reacting to another person's good news by showing authentic support and asking positive questions

Adaptation The ability to adjust to new information and experiences

Adaptive systems The cognitive (mental) and behavioral processes that allow people to adjust well to new information and experiences. Examples are problem-solving, motivation to learn new skills, development of strong and secure relationships, and cultural traditions

Affect The observable expression of emotions or feelings

Behavioral health The mental and emotional aspects of wellness, in addition to habits, substance use and abuse, and ways of expressing mental and emotional states through actions

Capitalization The act of sharing personal positive news with another

Cognitive behavioral therapy A form of psychological treatment that helps people see the relationship between beliefs, thoughts, and emotions, and resulting behavior patterns and actions. The assumption is that by adjusting our perceptions, we can directly influence our emotions and behaviors to be more productive

Collective efficacy People's ability to work collaboratively and effectively together for a common good

Compassion satisfaction Pleasure derived from being able to help those who are suffering

Compassion fatigue Secondary work-related trauma resulting from helping those who are in distress. It tends to result in a decrease in compassion over time

Coping How one faces and deals with responsibilities, problems, and stresses. **Active or approach coping**—Using one's own resources to recognize and deal with a situation, by seeking solutions to problems or seeking help from others, for example. **Avoidant coping**—Dealing with a problem by denying, ignoring or trying to get away from it. Usually results in behaviors that encourage distracting one's focus from the situation at hand, such as substance abuse, excessive sleeping, or withdrawal from others

Coping self-efficacy A belief in one's own ability to handle and deal effectively with the responsibilities, problems, and stresses that arise

Eudaimonia Virtuous living and fulfillment of human potential and excellence as characterized by the Greek philosopher Aristotle

Eudaimonic well-being Satisfaction from cultivating the best in oneself and realizing a deeper purpose and meaning in life

Hedonic well-being Pleasure, positive emotions, self-gratification, and the absence of pain and distress

Intervention Action performed with the intention of bringing about change

Learned helplessness A state brought on by the perception of not being able to control a situation and the belief that one's actions to try to exert control do not make a difference. It expresses itself as depression and passivity

Learned optimism Mastering the ability to interpret situations positively, disputing pessimistic thoughts when appropriate

Negative self-appraisal Unfavorable evaluations about oneself or how one performs in a situation

Mediator A variable that explains the relationship between two other variables. For example, coping self-efficacy mediates the relationship between a stressful situation and the development of psychological distress

Mindset How one thinks about things; the beliefs and expectations that shape one's reality and through which one filters experiences

Moderator A variable that influences the strength of the relationship between two other variables. For example, social support is a protective factor that moderates the relationship between an adverse situation and a resilient response

Motivation The desire or willingness to do something. **Intrinsic motivation**—Behavior driven by enjoyment of the activity itself. **Extrinsic motivation**—Behavior driven by external rewards such as money or fame

Optimism Confidence and hopefulness about the success of future outcomes. **Dispositional optimism**—Hopefulness about future events and believing that things can change for the better. **Realistic (or flexible) optimism**—Maintaining hopefulness within the constraints of what is true in a specific situation

Perceived prosocial impact The belief and judgment that one's actions are helpful to others

Positive psychology A field of scientific study into the mechanisms of positive human emotions and strengths, with a focus on the application and measurement of interventions to increase well-being, life satisfaction, physical health, and other conditions that lead to human thriving

Post-traumatic growth The experience of positive psychological change and transformation as the result of struggling with traumatic life situations

Prevention The action of stopping something from happening. **Primary prevention**—Stopping something undesirable from happening in the first place. **Secondary prevention**—Reducing the impact of an undesirable event that has already occurred to minimize adverse reactions. **Tertiary prevention**—Alleviating negative long-term effects of an undesirable situation that has already occurred and produced a lasting adverse reaction

Prosocial behavior Actions intended to benefit others

Reliability Repeatability and consistency of results of an approach or measure upon repeated application

Resilience The process of adapting in a positive way during or after stressful situations that involve adversity or risk

Self-efficacy The belief and confidence in one's ability to act in a way that brings about a desired outcome

Stress paradox The fact that stress can lead to both good and bad effects

Stress reappraisal Reinterpreting emotions, thoughts, and physical expressions of a stressful situation in a way that changes one's mindset about stress from negative to positive

Validity The degree to which an instrument or approach measures what it intends to measure

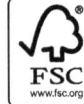

MIX
Papier aus verantwortungsvollen Quellen
Paper from responsible sources
FSC® C105338

If you have any concerns about our products,
you can contact us on
ProductSafety@springernature.com

In case Publisher is established outside the EU,
the EU authorized representative is:
**Springer Nature Customer Service Center GmbH
Europaplatz 3, 69115 Heidelberg, Germany**

Printed by Libri Plureos GmbH
in Hamburg, Germany